PHARMACOLOGY – RESEARCH, SAFETY TESTING AND REGULATION

# THE PHARMACOLOGICAL GUIDE TO PHENYTOIN

# Pharmacology – Research, Safety Testing and Regulation

Additional books and e-books in this series can be found on Nova's website under the Series tab.

PHARMACOLOGY – RESEARCH, SAFETY TESTING AND REGULATION

# THE PHARMACOLOGICAL GUIDE TO PHENYTOIN

PAYAL SUD
EDITOR

nova
Medicine & Health
New York

## Library of Congress Cataloging-in-Publication Data

Names: Sud, Payal, editor.
Title: The pharmacological guide to phenytoin / [edited by Payal Sud].
Description: New York : Nova Science Publishers, Inc., [2019] | Series: Pharmacology -- research, safety testing and regulation | Includes bibliographical references and index.
Identifiers: LCCN 2019058184 (print) | LCCN 2019058185 (ebook) | ISBN 9781536169805 (hardcover) | ISBN 9781536170146 (adobe pdf)
Subjects: LCSH: Phenytoin.
Classification: LCC RM666.P58 P43 2019 (print) | LCC RM666.P58 (ebook) | DDC 615.7/84--dc23
LC record available at https://lccn.loc.gov/2019058184
LC ebook record available at https://lccn.loc.gov/2019058185

*Published by Nova Science Publishers, Inc. † New York*

# CONTENTS

# PREFACE

The Pharmacological Guide to Phenytoin is a multi-authored text geared towards clinicians and pharmacists who will be prescribing and handling phenytoin or fosphenytoin. Each chapter in this book has been diligently written and peer reviewed by scholars in medical toxicology, pharmacology and emergency medicine.

What makes this book special compared to others in this field is the level of detail and evidence-based literature supporting the text in each chapter. Each author has performed a rigorous investigation of all available literature in order to provide the most up-to-date information and recommendations in each chapter.

We begin our journey in this book by delving into the history of phenytoin and fosphenytoin. After that, we establish guidelines for the administration, dosing and storage of the two drugs. These guidelines are supported by several previously published guidelines and landmark case reports. Majority of clinical trials focus on adults, and several studies utilize healthy, adult volunteers. Thus there is often scarce data on special populations such as pediatrics and patients with medical comorbidities. In the following chapter, we present how to manage phenytoin and fosphenytoin administration and toxicity in these populations.

After pharmacokinetics and toxicokinetics, we shift our focus to drug and food interactions. This chapter provides exquisite pharmacological detail on phenytoin and fosphenytoin, as well as their interactions with multiple xenobiotics. Having access to this knowledge will aid the clinician in the management of patients on these medications in various clinical scenarios, including multiple comorbidities, coingestants and environmental exposures. Discussing the toxicological profile of phenytoin and fosphenytoin is perhaps the most interesting section of this book. As with most available medical toxicology literature, given the paucity of randomized controlled trials, emphasis is placed on case reports. Finally, we discuss the diagnosis and management of phenytoin toxicity. The clinical manifestations of toxicity can mimic other medical emergencies, and with the knowledge and tools described clinicians can diagnose and treat their patients effectively.

The authors and I hope you find the information presented in this book educational as well as helpful in your practice, thus promoting the highest level of care to our patients.

Chapter 1 - The history of phenytoin starts with a shelved product developed in 1908 as a barbiturate derivative, which was believed to be of no clinical value at the time. It was not until 1923 that its potential as an epileptic was discovered. After much study, in 1976, Dilantin ® was approved by the FDA for the treatment of epilepsy. In order to prevent some of the side effects associated with phenytoin, a more water-soluble prodrug, fosphenytoin was developed and approved by the FDA in 2001. In addition to its use as an antiepileptic, phenytoin has been used in the past as a treatment for tricyclic antidepressant and digoxin toxicity, although it has fallen out of favor for those indications. Still a common drug in our epilepsy armamentarium, new advances in knowledge of this drug make it a potential treatment in wound healing and breast cancer.

Chapter 2 - Phenytoin, a hydantoin derivative, has several important pharmacotherapeutic implications and remains a cornerstone in the treatment of many seizure disorders. Although an important medication in several disease states, phenytoin can be potentially fatal in toxic concentrations and a thorough understanding of phenytoin's pharmacodynamics and pharmacokinetics is imperative to prevent patient morbidity and mortality. This chapter will discuss the multitude of indications for phenytoin, including its FDA approved indications as well as "off-label" therapeutic indications. Phenytoin is commercially available in several formulations including: chewable oral tablet, oral capsule, solution for injection (as sodium), and oral suspension; each of these administration routes will be discussed thoroughly. A large focus will be on the risks associated particularly with IV administration of both phenytoin and fosphenytoin (the water-soluble prodrug of phenytoin). Specifically, this chapter will describe the proposed mechanisms surrounding phenytoin/fosphenytoin induced extravasation and the more severe manifestation of extravasation, purple-glove syndrome (PGS). Following this discussion, we will delve into why fosphenytoin has a lower incidence of local cutaneous reactions and the treatments (both pharmacological and non-pharmacological) that clinicians should implement if the patient experiences such signs and symptoms consistent with ischemic progression of the affected distal extremity. In addition, this chapter will outline the appropriate storage conditions for phenytoin as to maintain appropriate potency/therapeutic effect and prevent degradation of its active and inactive ingredients. This chapter also goes into detail with a comprehensive discussion on the appropriate monitoring of phenytoin and when it is clinically indicated to draw serum phenytoin levels. Drawing serum phenytoin levels are important to guide therapeutic efficacy as well as determining the degree of toxicity in the acute or chronic overdose patient; interpreting these results and subsequently titrating the dose based on the measured serum levels are reviewed in depth in this chapter. Special populations are discussed, including those patients with low serum albumin levels (hypoalbuminemia) as well as patients with renal failure as this will significantly affect phenytoin's pharmacokinetics. Finally, this chapter will conclude with a brief discussion on switching between phenytoin's many different formulations.

Chapter 3 - This chapter will consider selected populations that require special attention with regards to the administration of phenytoin. It is important for clinicians to be aware of the variables at play that make these populations unique in order for therapy to be tailored thus avoiding toxicity. The neonatal and pediatric populations will be the focus, with some remarks on patients with liver and/or kidney impairment. This chapter will focus primarily on the alterations of the pharmacokinetics in these populations since most of the susceptibility to toxicity are due to these differences. Differences in the pharmacokinetics of these populations as compared to the general population requires caution and special attention to dosing, drug level monitoring, focused history and examination, and the recognition/management of toxicity.

Preceding the highlights of special considerations in the neonatal and pediatric populations will be a discussion on phenytoin's historical and present role in the management of childhood epilepsy. Trends in phenytoin's use as compared to other traditional antiepileptic drugs (AEDs) will be discussed in the context of the available literature. Focus will turn to the general physiological and pharmacological differences between the neonatal/pediatric populations as compared to the general population. This will highlight important principles necessary to understand how some of these differences pertain specifically to the administration of phenytoin in these populations. Age dependent adverse effects will be explored with regards to differences in incidence and presentation in these populations. Finally, special consideration relating to the history, physical and management primarily pertaining to the evaluation of phenytoin toxicity will be considered.

A vast majority of medications are affected by alterations in hepatic and renal function. Phenytoin is a classic example of how impairments in either the liver or kidneys can dramatically alter phenytoin concentrations predisposing these populations at increased risk for toxicity.

Unfortunately, evidence-based research is often scarce and limited in these special populations. This is not only true of phenytoin but a common limitation in the evaluation and understanding of many medications that are commonly used in these populations. Very few randomized trials are available in support of the information contained in this chapter. Rather, literature will often be dependent on available observational and case reports/series studies. While limitations in available literature is common, this chapter will provide information valuable to the health care provider in order to make cognizant decisions and recommendations to patients in these special populations.

Chapter 4 - Phenytoin is a barbiturate derivative used primarily for its non-sedating anti-epileptic properties and commonly as a second line agent in status epilepticus. It is highly protein bound and its clinical effect is determined by the concentration of free unbound phenytoin. It demonstrates saturable nonlinear metabolism and has a narrow therapeutic index. Additionally, there is a wide inter-individual variability in clinical response to dosage that can be attributed to genetic variations in metabolism. These factors make it impossible to generalize dosing regimens. Patients on maintenance therapy with phenytoin must have their dosages individualized with monitoring of serum phenytoin concentration until a steady state can be established. While general ranges of a safe therapeutic serum concentration have been established from studies as early as the 1960s, understanding the pharmacokinetics of phenytoin may help underscore the importance of individualized drug monitoring and may aid in recognizing the multitude of factors that may lead to toxicity or under treatment. Fosphenytoin is a prodrug of phenytoin that was developed as a safer alternative to intravenous phenytoin but it has its own unique considerations and side effects will also be discussed.

Chapter 5 - Phenytoin is an antiepileptic drug that displays complex pharmacokinetic characteristics. These unique characteristics result in clinically important interactions with other drugs as well as food and nutrients. In addition to being responsible for causing a significant number of drug interactions, phenytoin metabolism may also be adversely impacted by a large amount of drugs. The clinical implications of these interactions can place patients at increased risk for phenytoin toxicity and adverse events, or alternately may result in a subtherapeutic response which can precipitate seizures and result in drug therapy failure.

This chapter will review the mechanisms and consequences of phenytoin related drug-drug and drug-nutrient interactions.

Chapter 6 - Toxicity from phenytoin overdose is dependent on the route of administration, duration of exposure (acute and chronic), and the dosage. Phenytoin is found in both oral and intravenous formulations and is also available as a water-soluble prodrug, fosphenytoin. Toxicity is manifested when serum levels exceed the therapeutic level, leading to classic cerebellar and vestibular dysfunction with symptoms such as nystagmus, slurred speech, and ataxia. In addition, phenytoin also produces toxicity through the cardiovascular system, gastrointestinal system, skin, gums, hematopoietic system, and liver.

Chapter 7 - Phenytoin is a widely used antiepileptic medications and considered the first line treatment in most seizure disorders. With its popular use in the population, the ability to detect and manage its toxicity are important skills for all physicians. Although concentrations of the drug are available through laboratory analysis, the physician must have a high index of suspicion first, as the physician needs to know when to send the sample for analysis. Certain physical exam findings can assist in determining if toxicity is present. In addition to overdose, the Purple Glove Syndrome is one specific adverse effect of phenytoin that must be considered and discussed, which has decreased in incidence since the development of a more water-soluble prodrug fosphenytoin. Once the diagnosis of toxicity is established, the treatment remains largely supportive, with hemodynamic, respiratory, mental status and neurologic monitoring. Deaths are rare, even after massive overdoses. Multi dose activated charcoal (MDAC) can enhance clearance of the drug from the body, with questionable effect on the clinical manifestations. There is a limited role for extracorporeal treatments in phenytoin toxicity, with specific recommendations and guidelines established. Disposition depends on the clinical scenario, with frequent neurological assessments required in those displaying neurotoxicity. Cardiotoxicity typically only occurs with intravenous (IV) phenytoin and requires cardiac monitoring, but this rarely occurs after an oral overdose.

In: The Pharmacological Guide to Phenytoin ISBN: 978-1-53616-980-5
Editor: Payal Sud 

*Chapter 1*

# The History of Phenytoin

***Maria F. Escarcia*[1], *D.O. and Angela Regina*[2,*], *D.O.***
[1]Department of Emergency Medicine, St. Barnabas Health System, Bronx, NY, US
[2]Department of Emergency Medicine and Medical Toxicology, St. Barnabas Health System, Bronx, NY, US

## Abstract

The history of phenytoin starts with a shelved product developed in 1908 as a barbiturate derivative, which was believed to be of no clinical value at the time. It was not until 1923 that its potential as an epileptic was discovered. After much study, in 1976, Dilantin ® was approved by the FDA for the treatment of epilepsy. In order to prevent some of the side effects associated with phenytoin, a more water-soluble prodrug, fosphenytoin was developed and approved by the FDA in 2001. In addition to its use as an antiepileptic, phenytoin has been used in the past as a treatment for tricyclic antidepressant and digoxin toxicity, although it has fallen out of favor for those indications. Still a common drug in our epilepsy armamentarium, new advances in knowledge of this drug make it a potential treatment in wound healing and breast cancer.

* Corresponding Author's Email: areginatox@gmail.com.

## Introduction

Prior to the development of phenytoin, antiepileptic medications were sedating. The search for a non-sedating medication for the treatment of seizures started in 1908, with a drug that for years was not believed to have any clinical utility. After years of study, it was approved in 1976 under the brand name Dilantin®. Since its approval, phenytoin has had an interesting history including use in various fields of medicine including cardiology and toxicology. In 2001 a more water soluble prodrug was developed in response to side effects with the intravenous formulation of phenytoin.

## The History of Antiepileptics

Epilepsy is a condition as old as mankind, though the first mention of seizure activity in text wasn't until 2000 B.C. The condition was written about in an ancient Mesopotamian language and the disease was termed *antasubbû*, which was thought to be brought on by the god of the moon and translates to "the hand of sin." Babylonians also make mention of epilepsy in *The Sakikku*, one of the oldest Babylonian medical texts. The use of the term *antasubba,* was an all-encompassing term for all seizure types. In early Babylon, Antasubba was attributed to evil spirits and the ancient Greeks believed epilepsy to be a divine punishment for sinners [1]. Given the mysticism that shrouded the medical condition, initial treatments consisted of mainly a means to ward off the disease. Remedies and amulets were widely used in the treatment and prophylaxis of epileptic events. In colonial days, amulets of peony root, coral, mistletoe or grey hound dog hair were used as a means to protect against seizures. Vigorous exercise was also highly encouraged [2]. In 1799, John Bostock, a Liverpool physician, reported his findings of silver nitrate, in the management of epilepsy. The report describes successful seizure control in a young shoemaker using one fifth of a gram of silver nitrate taken daily along with Peruvian tree bark. The patient was described as an 11-year-old boy with history of new onset seizures that had gradually progressed from affecting him once daily, to approximately five times per day. Within approximately one month of starting the medication the patient was described as seizure free [3]. Although seemingly effective, this treatment carried a high risk of toxicity and development of argyria, which is an irreversible blue discoloration to the skin seen with chronic silver ingestion [2].

Potassium bromide is considered the first medication to start the repertoire of antiepileptic drugs. It made its debut as an antiepileptic treatment in the English medical journal, The Lancet in 1857 by mention of Sir Charles Locock [4]. Sir Charles Locock, a London physician, became an elected fellow of the Royal College of Physicians in 1836 and also served as a member of the Royal College of Physicians Council from 1840-1842 [5]. Locock served as president of the Royal Medical and Chirurgical society in 1857 and was also appointed as the personal obstetrician to Queen Victoria [4, 5]. In 1857, Sir Charles Locock chaired a meeting of the Royal Medical and Chirurgical society at which Sir Edward Sieveking presented an analysis of 52 cases of epilepsy. Following Sieveking's presentation, Locock made a concluding response. Locock described cases of "infantile epilepsy related to dentition," "epilepsy due to sexual indulgence" and "hysterical epilepsy" which were not previously mentioned in the earlier case analysis given by Sieveking. Locock believed in a correlation between sexual excitement and menstruation as a trigger for epilepsy, termed catamenial epilepsy. In his concluding remarks he mentions a recent report of several men experiencing reversible impotence while taking potassium bromide. Locock thus, used this reasoning for prescribing potassium bromide to women in order to suppress seizure activity by means of repressing their sexual drive. Locock also reported his observations in successfully treating 13 out of 14 cases of catamenial epilepsy with potassium bromide during that meeting [5]. From then on bromide salts remained a mainstay in the treatment of epilepsy until the 20$^{th}$ century. Some of the difficulties encountered with bromide salts were their high toxicity, long half-life and ability to accumulate in tissues. Therefore, when phenobarbital was introduced into the market, bromide salts were phased out of favor for the treatment of epilepsy [6].

The origin of phenobarbital begins with the introduction of the benzene ring. German chemist, Agust Kekulé, mused during a meeting of the German Chemical Society that the ring structure of benzene came to him in a dream [7]. The structure of the benzene ring was first published by Agust Kekulé, in 1865. Barbituric acid was first developed in 1864 by German chemist, Adolf von Baeyer [7, 8]. There is some speculation as to how the compound came to be named. Some hypothesized that the chemical compound was synthesized on December 4$^{th}$ 1864, which is a day known as The Feast of Saint Barbara in the Eastern Orthodox and Catholic churches. Others hypothesized the compound was derived using the urine of an acquaintance of his named Barbara [7]. Conrad Guthzeit subsequently synthesized diethylbarbituric acid, a member of the barbiturate family, in 1881 by using barbituric acid in conjunction with ethyl iodide [6].

However, it wasn't until 1903 that diethylbarbituric acid was used medicinally. It was noted by Emil Fischer, a Noble Prize winner in Chemistry in 1902, and Joseph von Mering, a pharmacology professor at the University of Halle, that the medication exhibited a hypnotic or sleep-inducing effect in dogs [6, 7]. Fischer and Mering also reported a relationship between the hypnotic activity and the structure of some urea-containing compounds and urea derivatives. This relationship led to their hypothesis that diethylbarbituric acid could serve as a clinically useful hypnotic [8]. The pharmaceutical company Bayer soon began manufacturing the drug under the trade name Veronal®. The drug has been said to be named by Mering, after the Italian city of Verona, the most peaceful town he had visited [6, 7]. Other authors argue that the name Veronal stems from the latin word *verus*, meaning true, as it was claimed to be the "true" hypnotic by Fisher [6]. After the United States entered into World War I, Congress passed the Trading with the Enemy Act of 1917, which allowed for manufacturing of German products protected by patent, under the conditions that the generic name be modified and the profits be allotted to the American Subsidiaries of the German companies. Via these rules, diethylbarbituric acid was renamed Barbital in the United States. As a result of a similar regulation in the United Kingdom, diethylbarbituric acid became known as Barbitone in the United Kingdom [6].

With slight modifications to the barbituric acid molecule, more than 2,500 different barbiturate derivatives were synthesized by 1960 [6, 7]. However, of the thousands of compounds synthesized, only about 50 made it onto the market and only a few dozen were habitually used in the clinical setting [6]. In an attempt to find a more stable hypnotic, Heinrich Höerlein produced one of the most widely used barbiturates in 1911. He altered the original structure of the barbituric ring by substituting a phenyl radical for one of the two ethyl radicals, resulting in 5,5-phenylethylbarbituric acid (aka: phenobarbital or Luminal®) [8]. Phenobarbital was first used in therapy as a hypnotic agent in 1912 and was commercialized that same year with the name Luminal® by F. Bayer and company [6]. Phenobarbital's longer duration of action compared to barbital allowed it to become the hypnotic of choice in hospitals as well as in outpatient care [6].

Phenobarbital's antiepileptic utility was first reported by Alfred Hauptmann, a resident psychiatrist in Freiburg Germany, on February 1912. Hauptmann slept over an epilepsy ward and was constantly awakened by the sound of seizing patients. He began administering phenobarbital at nighttime and noted that not only did the patient have fewer seizures during the night, but also remained seizure free the following morning [6, 7]. Hauptmann proceeded to record his findings and later began to systematically examine phenobarbital as an antiepileptic treatment [7]. One of the most notable deductions made by Hauptmann was phenobarbital's ability to reduce both seizure frequency and intensity, which allowed patient to lead a more normal life [6]. Hauptmann also reported having chosen phenobarbital, a known hypnotic, to test as an antiepileptic particularly because of its sedating qualities [8]. Unfortunately, phenobarbital's international debut as an antiepileptic was delayed, due in part to Hauptmann publishing his findings in a small journal that was not well known internationally and also due to World War I [6]. It wasn't until the late 1920's that phenobarbital largely displaced bromides as the mainstay in epilepsy treatment [8].

## History of Phenytoin

Phenytoin, also known as 5,5-diphenylimidazolidine-2,4-dione or diphenylhydantoin is a molecule first synthesized by Henrich Biltz in 1908 at the University of Kiel, Germany. Initially the compound sparked little interest in the pharmaceutical world as it did not exhibit much hypnotic activity. It wasn't until 1923 that it was resynthesized by Arthur Dox at Parke-Davis Pharmaceutical Company in the United States. The compound, a phenobarbital analog, was resynthesized in the hopes of finding a new hypnotic medication for the treatment of epilepsy.[9] As previously mentioned, during this time bromide salts and phenobarbital were the treatment of choice, and both of these medications were highly sedating. It was assumed by scientists at the time that the hypnotic activity was responsible for their anticonvulsive effects.[2] Diphenylhydantoin has two phenyl rings at the C5 position of the hydantoin molecule, making it a non-sedating anticonvulsant [10]. Because of its non-hypnotic effects, the molecule was deemed "inactive" and shelved in the lab for over 10 years [9].

### The Boston City Hospital Neurology Team

Tracy Putnam and H. Houston Merritt began working together in 1935 at the Boston City Hospital Neurological unit, along with other brilliant minds that made countless contributions to the study of epilepsy [8]. The Boston City Hospital neurologic team was established by Dr. Stanley Cobb in 1922, after being appointed director of the neurologic unit [8, 9]. Cobb's team included Dr. William Lennox, a long-standing humanitarian; nationally and abroad. Lennox also established the Seizure Unit at Boston Children's Hospital. A form of childhood epilepsy, Lennox-Gastaut syndrome, was named in honor of Dr. Lennox along with Dr. Henri Gastaut for the strides made by the two physicians in the field of epilepsy [9]. Dr. Lennox, in the following years, came to be known as the "father of epileptology" and as the "father in the fight against epilepsy" [8]. Erna

Leonhardt, initially hired as a technician, quickly became a contributor to their research and an integral part of the team [8, 9]. Leonhardt went on to marry Dr. Frederic Gibbs in 1930, who joined the team after graduating from Johns Hopkins Medical School [8, 9]. The Gibbs were some of the first to advance the use electroencephalographic (EEG) technique and refine it as a research and clinical instrument [8]. Dr. Gibbs also headed the first electroencephalographic lab in the world. Dr. Tracy J. Putnam was a Boston Brahmin, whose father was a renowned professor of neurologic disease at Harvard Medical School [8]. Putnam graduated from Harvard Medical School and went on to conduct research in the field of neurosurgery for a year in Europe. Upon returning to Boston, Putnam trained in neurosurgery under Dr. Harvey Cushing; he also trained in the field of neurology under Dr. Cobb [9]. When Cobb became head of the neurology unit at the Boston City Hospital, Putnam was given a formal research position in both fields of neurology and neurosurgery [8, 9]. H. Houston Merritt graduated from Johns Hopkins Medical School. He completed his internship at Yale and subsequently became a neurology resident at the Boston City Hospital. Upon graduating from residency Merritt joined Harvard as medical faculty and also joined Cobb's neurologic research unit [8, 9]. In 1934 Putnam took over Cobbs position as head of the Neurology Unit when Cobb took a position at Massachusetts General Hospital [9]. This prestigious team of physicians and scientists whose main interest of study was epilepsy created a nurturing environment where ideas and research could flourish. The Boston City Hospital neurology group was said be comprised of a relatively liberal setting in which the team was receptive to bold ideas, and placed a high priority on intellect and free exchange of ideas [8].

While working at the Boston City Hospital, Putnam and Merritt attended a presentation for the American Society for Clinical Investigation, given by Dr. Tinsley Harrison. Dr. Harrison is famously known within the medical community for authoring Principles of Internal Medicine. Harrison shared that elevated concentrations of conjugated phenols, which are seen in renal failure patients, appeared to produce a motor depressant effect. According to the presentation, this finding was the reason that this patient population did not exhibit convulsions that would otherwise occur [8, 9]. This prompted

Putnam and Merritt to study phenyl derivatives as other possible antiepileptics. They contacted multiple pharmaceutical companies, including Parke-Davis, who sent multiple barbiturate analogs, one of which was diphenylhydantoin.

## Animal Studies

As far back as the late 1800s it was known that abnormal neuronal electrical discharges triggered seizure activity [2]. Putnam, also having worked closely with Dr. Frederick Gibbs, who headed the first electroencephalographic laboratory in the world, stated in one of his papers "every true seizure is attended by an electrical storm in the brain" [8]. Having this knowledge, Putnam and Merritt, with the help of Frederick Gibbs and Paul Hoefer, developed a method to test these phenyl derivatives on animals. Together, they developed a systematic approach to screen the anticonvulsive compounds.

The cats were placed in a restraining box and electrodes were placed on the scalp, between the ears in a shaven area, and in the mouth. A pulsed current, provided by a 45V battery, was interrupted 80 times per second and was administered via the scalp-mouth electrodes. A millimeter was used to measure the amount of current passing through the cat's brain [2]. The current was steadily applied for 10 seconds and was increased at 5-minute intervals until the cat exhibited a tonic-clonic seizure. The amount of current required to produce a seizure was recorded, measured in milliamperes, and used as the control convulsive threshold for that particular cat. The test drug was then administered orally to the same animal and after approximately 2-3 hours the aforementioned steps were repeated until a seizure occurred. Each drug was then ranked based on the amount of elevation in convulsive threshold. A rating of '0' meant the convulsive threshold was not affected, a '+' equated an elevation in convulsive threshold of 5-15 mA, a '2+' equated an elevation of convulsive threshold of 20-30 mA, a '3+' indicated an elevation in convulsive threshold up to 50 mA and a '4+' indicated an elevation in convulsive threshold greater than

50 mA. Initial findings demonstrated that an oral dose of sodium bromide, enough to prevent a cat from walking, elevated the cat's convulsive threshold by 50 percent. Phenobarbital administered orally, again in a dose high enough to prevent the cat from walking, elevated the convulsive threshold by 300-400%. With phenobarbital performing significantly better than sodium bromide, Putnam began to question the previous notion of hypnotic qualities as a requirement for an efficacious antiepileptic. When he tested diphenylhydantoin, an effective, non-sedating antiepileptic drug was discovered [2]. Diphenylhydantoin, acetophenone and benzophenone, were found to have the greatest separation between anticonvulsant efficacy and hypnotic activity [9, 10].

Diphenylhydantoin was then chosen for further clinical investigation. Although it is difficult to ascertain why this drug in particular was chosen it is likely because it subjectively seemed to cause the least degree of toxicity [8]. The compound was prepared as a sodium salt as it allowed for better solubility [9, 10]. Clinical trials began in May 1937 and the first report of their findings was one year later in June 1938 before the Section on Nervous and Mental Diseases of the American Medical Association. The findings confirmed the observations in the preliminary animal studies [9]. In a follow up presentation, Putnam and Merrit reported that sodium diphenylhydantoinate was most effective in controlling psychomotor seizures, second most effective in preventing grand mal seizures and least effective in preventing petit mal seizures [8]. The medication became a marketed drug in 1938 as Sodium Diphenylhydantoin or Dilantin®, and in that same year also began clinical trials on children [9]. The following year the American Medical Association Council on Pharmacy and Chemistry added Dilantin® to its drug compendium. The medication was intended for epileptic patients refractory to phenobarbital or bromides or for those whose medications produced disagreeable side effects [8]. In the initial clinical trials, Putnam and Merritt observed some of the medication's side effects such as rash, ataxia and gingival hyperplasia, however it wasn't until decades later that teratogenicity and fetal hydantoin syndrome were noted [9].

## PHENYTOIN AND ITS PRODRUG: FOSPHENYTOIN

Currently, phenytoin is available in both oral and intravenous formulations. There are various clinical circumstances in which an intravenous administration may be preferred over oral. For example, patients that are non-compliant with medications, patients with low serum phenytoin concentrations and those who for various reasons cannot take medications orally. In some instances, intramuscular administration might be preferred or required, such as when intravenous access is difficult to obtain or catheter size is smaller than 20-gauge [11]. Phenytoin sodium, however can have some less than desirable side effects and administration issues when administered intravenously and intramuscularly. For this reason, a prodrug of phenytoin; fosphenytoin or Cerebyx®, was developed to aid in the safety and efficacy of parenteral phenytoin administration.

Phenytoin sodium has limited aqueous solubility and because of this the intravenous formulations consist of an aqueous vehicle of 40% propylene glycol and 10% alcohol with a pH of 12. This alkaline pH is required as phenytoin exhibits poor solubility at a lower pH. Intravenous administration can be painful or irritating and has the potential to cause soft tissue injury if it infiltrates the soft tissue [12]. Unfortunately, dilution of phenytoin sodium to minimize these undesired effects causes the solution to precipitate which can lead to crystallization and phlebitis. Intramuscular administration is also very painful and results in slow, unpredictable absorption [11, 12].

Fosphenytoin or Cerebyx® was developed in 1997 as a water-soluble prodrug of phenytoin that can be administered intramuscularly and intravenously [13]. Fosphenytoin is a phosphate ester derivative of phenytoin sodium and is indicated for the control of generalized convulsive status epilepticus and to prevent and treat seizures during neurosurgery [11, 12]. Fosphenytoin is measured in phenytoin sodium equivalents (PE). The prodrug is 4,400 times more soluble than its predecessor. The medication is supplied as a ready mixed solution in water containing buffer additives, giving it a pH ranging from 8.6-9.0.

Fosphenytoin is metabolized by phosphatases found in blood and tissue into phenytoin sodium, along with phosphate and formate [12]. Half-life of conversion from fosphenytoin to phenytoin sodium is approximately 8 15 minutes. Bioavailability of the phenytoin converted from both intravenous and intramuscular fosphenytoin is 100% [12, 13]. Fosphenytoin has no intrinsic activity prior to its conversion to phenytoin sodium and also does not exhibit any side effects in addition to those for which phenytoin is responsible for. IV fosphenytoin, however is approximately 18 times more costly than IV phenytoin. The average wholesale price for 500mg of IV phenytoin is $4.10 vs $73.36 for 500mg IV fosphenytoin [11]. Although individual cost analysis may show this relative cost discrepancy to be significantly less as additional cost is acquired when treating the many complications of parenteral phenytoin administration.

## More Uses

Since its discovery, phenytoin has demonstrated multiple modes of action and thus has been used to treat conditions other than epilepsy over the years. Most notably, phenytoin is both a sodium channel and calcium channel antagonist and is thus characterized as a broad acting ion channel antagonist [10]. This mechanism is not only responsible for its antiepileptic effects, but also for its use as an antiarrhythmic. Phenytoin is categorized as a class IB antiarrhythmic, although it is not widely employed for this use due to its side effect profile.

Phenytoin has been shown to have clinical utility in patients with tricyclic antidepressant (TCA) cardiotoxicity that are refractory to sodium bicarbonate and hypertonic saline. Although there are no randomized control trials, a small case series found low doses (5-7 mg/kg) of IV phenytoin given to patient exhibiting TCA cardiotoxicity normalized PRI and QRS duration. 50% of subjects exhibited PRI and QRS normalization within 46 minutes, while the remaining 50% achieved normalization of PRI and QRS within 14 hours of presentation to the emergency department [14]. Another small prospective study administered phenytoin to seven patients with QRS widening (greater than 100 ms), three of whom had ventricular arrhythmias. 100% of patients exhibited a decrease in QRS by 55 ± 25% from patient's baseline and in each of the three cases of ventricular arrhythmias, QRS normalized during phenytoin administration [12].

Phenytoin has also proved to be useful in cases of digoxin toxicity secondary to an acute overdose. The use of this medication in digitalis toxicity was first proposed in the 1950s. Phenytoin is a negative ionotropic agent, it improves AV conduction, and suppresses digoxin induced ventricular automaticity [15]. Repeated doses of phenytoin have been shown to ameliorate blocks in AV conduction which results in a greater atrial input to the ventricle. One case report in 1974 demonstrated the usefulness of repeated low doses of phenytoin administered early in the treatment of acute digitalis overdose with a successful outcome [15]. However, the use of phenytoin has fallen out of favor in the setting of digitalis toxicity since the introduction of Digoxin immune fab.

The field of dermatology has also employed a use for phenytoin. Phenytoin demonstrated inhibition of collagenase and has been studied for the use of wound healing, connective tissue diseases and other dermatologic inflammatory processes [10]. Gingival hyperplasia is a well-known side effect of phenytoin. It was first reported in 1938, one year after phenytoin was introduced into the market [16]. This side effect lead scientists to investigate which property of the medication was causing this effect and how it could be used in the field of wound healing and connective tissue disorders. In the late 1950s it was observed that non-epileptic patients with experimentally induced gingival ulcers experienced increased rates of healing [16]. In 1958, Pathologists from the Indiana University School of Medicine conducted a controlled experimental study on the effect of phenytoin on the tensile strength of healing wounds. They administered 50mg of phenytoin orally to rats. The results demonstrated a significant increase in the tensile strength in healing wounds on rats [16]. The findings in this study triggered more research and randomized controlled trials in dermatologic disorders, including mucositis, wound healing, vitiligo, burns and dystrophic epidermolysis bullosa. In 2007 a systemic review of 14 randomized controlled trials in this field concluded that phenytoin may have a positive effect on wound healing, but the studies are deemed to be of intermediate quality. Unfortunately, too many unstudied variables remain this this field [16].

Most recently, in 2015, phenytoin was discovered to have a strong affinity for estrogen alpha receptors and is currently being studied in its effects on breast cancer [10]. A study in 2015 found that phenytoin, at clinically effective concentrations, acts as a strong estrogen receptor alpha cell antagonist and also as a many-fold weaker agonist [17]. Phenytoin binds to the estrogen alpha receptor at the hinge of helix 12 and can potentially interfere with the entry of other estrogen receptor ligands and with the mobility of helix 12. Phenytoin did not appear to have an effect on cells that only contained estrogen beta receptors [17]. These findings opened the door for phenytoin as a potential estrogen modulator in the treatment of estrogen alpha receptor mediated diseases, such as in breast cancer. A different study conducted in 2012 evaluated phenytoin's effect on sodium current, invasion and migration of breast cancer cells. Voltage gated sodium channels are expressed in breast cancer cells and mediate action potential firing, neurite growth, pathfinding and migration. Phenytoin was found to inhibit transient and persistent sodium current from strongly metastatic breast cancer cells [18]. At a therapeutic concentration for treatment of epilepsy, phenytoin inhibited migration and invasion of metastatic breast cancer cells, but had no effect on weakly metastatic breast cancer cells, likely because they do not express sodium currents [18].

## CONCLUSION

Phenytoin is a drug that was initially believed to have no clinical utility. Its main indication is for epilepsy, but it has also been used for other conditions such as arrhythmia and toxicity from TCA and digoxin. Although no longer used for those conditions, new advances show potential for its use in wound healing and breast cancer. It is still a common antiepileptic, but only further time and study will show what the future holds for this drug which was initially shelved in 1908.

## REFERENCES

[1] Magiorkinis, Emmanouil, Kalliopi Sidiropoulou, and Aristidis Diamantis. "Hallmarks in the History of Epilepsy: Epilepsy in Antiquity." *Epilepsy & Behavior* 17, no. 1 (2010): 103-08. doi: 10. 1016/j.yebeh.2009.10.023.

[2] Glazko, Anthony J. "Discovery of Phenytoin." *Therapeutic Drug Monitoring* 8, no. 4 (1986): 490-97. doi: 10.1097/00007691-19861 2000-00021.

[3] Bostock, John. "Dr. Bostock, on the Nitrat of Silver, in Epilepsy." *The Medical and Physical Journal* 1, no. 3 (May 1799): 222-24. https://www.ncbi.nlm.nih.gov/pmc/articles/PMC5650772/.

[4] Brodie, Martin J. "Antiepileptic Drug Therapy the Story so Far." *Seizure* 19, no. 10 (2010): 650-55. doi: 10.1016/j.seizure.2010.10.027.

[5] Eadie, Mj. "Sir Charles Locock and Potassium Bromide." *The Journal of the Royal College of Physicians of Edinburgh* 42, no. 3 (2012): 274-79. doi: 10.4997/jrcpe.2012.317.

[6] López-Muñoz, F, R Ucha-Udabe, and C Alamo. "The History of Barbiturates a Century after Their Clinical Introduction." *Neuropsychiatric Disease and Treatment* 1, no. 4 (December 2005): 329–43.

[7] Yasiry, Zeid, and Simon D. Shorvon. "How Phenobarbital Revolutionized Epilepsy Therapy: The Story of Phenobarbital Therapy in Epilepsy in the Last 100 Years." *Epilepsia* 53 (2012): 26–39. https://doi.org/10.1111/epi.12026.

[8] Friedlander, Walter J. "Putnam, Merritt, and the Discovery of Dilantin®." *Epilepsia* 27, no. S3 (1986). doi: 10.1111/j.1528-1157. 1986.tb05743.x.

[9] Anderson, R. J. "The Little Compound That Could: How Phenytoin Changed Drug Discovery and Development." *Molecular Interventions* 9, no. 5 (October 01, 2009): 208-14. doi: 10.1124/ mi.9. 5.1.

[10] Hesselink, Jan M. Keppel, and David J. Kopsky. "Phenytoin: 80 years Young, from Epilepsy to Breast Cancer, a Remarkable Molecule with Multiple Modes of Action." *Journal of Neurology* 264, no. 8 (January 12, 2017): 1617-621. doi: 10.1007/s00415-017-8391-5.

[11] Lin, Tyrone. "Pharmacotherapy Update: Fosphenytoin (Cerebyx®)." *Pharmacotherapy Update | Fosphenytoin (Cerebyx®), 2005*. https://www.clevelandclinicmeded.com/medicalpubs/pharmacy/novdec2004/fosphenytoin.htm.

[12] Boucher, Bradley A. "Fosphenytoin: A Novel Phenytoin Prodrug." *Pharmacotherapy: The Journal of Human Pharmacology and Drug Therapy* 16, no. 5 (1996): 777–91. https://doi.org/10.1002/j.1875-9114.1996.tb02996.x.

[13] Hoffman, Robert Steven, Mary Ann. Howland, Neal A. Lewin, Lewis Nelson, Lewis R. Goldfrank, and Neal Flomenbaum. *Goldfranks Toxicologic Emergencies*. 10th ed. New York: McGraw-Hill, 2015.

[14] Foianini, Anthony, Timothy Joseph Wiegand, and Neal Benowitz. "What Is the Role of Lidocaine or Phenytoin in Tricyclic Antidepressant-induced Cardiotoxicity?" *Clinical Toxicology* 48, no. 4 (2010): 325-30. doi:10.3109/15563650.2010.487050.

[15] Rumack, B. H., R. R. Wolfe, and H. Gilfrich. "Phenytoin (diphenylhydantoin) Treatment of Massive Digoxin Overdose." *British Heart Journal* 36, no. 4 (1974): 405-08. doi: 10.1136/hrt. 36.4.405.

[16] Keppel Hesselink, Jan M. "Phenytoin Repositioned in Wound Healing: Clinical Experience Spanning 60 Years." *Drug Discovery Today* 23, no. 2 (October 6, 2017): 402–8. https://www.sciencedirect.com/science/article/pii/S135964461730096X.

[17] Fadiel, A, J Song, D Tivon, A Hamza, T Cardozo, and F Naftolin. "Phenytoin Is an Estrogen Receptor α-Selective Modulator That

Interacts With Helix 12." *Reproductive Sciences* 22, no. 2 (2015): 146–55. https://doi.org/ 10.1177/1933719114549853.

[18] Yang, Ming, David J. Kozminski, Lindsey A. Wold, Rohan Modak, Jeffrey D. Calhoun, Lori L. Isom, and William J. Brackenbury. "Therapeutic Potential for Phenytoin: Targeting Nav1.5 Sodium Channels to Reduce Migration and Invasion in Metastatic Breast Cancer." *Breast Cancer Research and Treatment* 134, no. 2 (August 2012): 603–15. https://doi.org/10.1007/s10549-012-2102-9.

In: The Pharmacological Guide to Phenytoin ISBN: 978-1-53616-980-5
Editor: Payal Sud 

*Chapter 2*

# CLINICAL INDICATIONS, DOSING AND DOSAGE FORMS: ADULTS

***William Heuser*[*], MS**
Department of Emergency Medicine,
Long Island Jewish Medical Center,
Northwell Health, New Hyde Park, NY, US

## ABSTRACT

Phenytoin, a hydantoin derivative, has several important pharmacotherapeutic implications and remains a cornerstone in the treatment of many seizure disorders. Although an important medication in several disease states, phenytoin can be potentially fatal in toxic concentrations and a thorough understanding of phenytoin's pharmacodynamics and pharmacokinetics is imperative to prevent patient morbidity and mortality. This chapter will discuss the multitude of indications for phenytoin, including its FDA approved indications as well as "off-label" therapeutic indications. Phenytoin is commercially available in several formulations including: chewable oral tablet, oral capsule, solution for injection (as sodium), and oral suspension; each of these

[*] Corresponding Author's Email: wheuser@northwell.edu.

administration routes will be discussed thoroughly. A large focus will be on the risks associated particularly with IV administration of both phenytoin and fosphenytoin (the water-soluble prodrug of phenytoin). Specifically, this chapter will describe the proposed mechanisms surrounding phenytoin/fosphenytoin induced extravasation and the more severe manifestation of extravasation, purple-glove syndrome (PGS). Following this discussion, we will delve into why fosphenytoin has a lower incidence of local cutaneous reactions and the treatments (both pharmacological and non-pharmacological) that clinicians should implement if the patient experiences such signs and symptoms consistent with ischemic progression of the affected distal extremity. In addition, this chapter will outline the appropriate storage conditions for phenytoin as to maintain appropriate potency/therapeutic effect and prevent degradation of its active and inactive ingredients. This chapter also goes into detail with a comprehensive discussion on the appropriate monitoring of phenytoin and when it is clinically indicated to draw serum phenytoin levels. Drawing serum phenytoin levels are important to guide therapeutic efficacy as well as determining the degree of toxicity in the acute or chronic overdose patient; interpreting these results and subsequently titrating the dose based on the measured serum levels are reviewed in depth in this chapter. Special populations are discussed, including those patients with low serum albumin levels (hypoalbuminemia) as well as patients with renal failure as this will significantly affect phenytoin's pharmacokinetics. Finally, this chapter will conclude with a brief discussion on switching between phenytoin's many different formulations.

## Indications for Use

### FDA-Approved Indications

Phenytoin has a multitude of indications based upon on its mechanism as a neuronal membrane stabilizer via inhibition (or increasing efflux) of sodium ions across cell membranes. FDA approved indications for phenytoin include, status epilepticus (injection only) and non-emergent seizures. In non-emergent seizures, Phenytoin is effective in controlling generalized tonic-clonic and complex partial (psychomotor, temporal lobe) seizures and also in the prevention and treatment of seizures occurring during or following neurosurgery).

## "Off-Label" Indications

Phenytoin also has "off-label" indications for the prevention of early (within 1 week) posttraumatic seizures following traumatic brain injury (Level of evidence A, G).

Additional "off-label" indications for phenytoin include its utility in mood stabilization in patients with bipolar affective disorder (current episode depression) as well as rapid cycling bipolar affective disorder. Phenytoin has also shown promising results in the treatment of neuropathic pain given its novel mechanism at the sodium channel.

Although most commonly used as an anticonvulsant to treat seizures, phenytoin has important implications as an effective treatment for polymorphic ventricular tachycardia due to QT prolongation, particularly in patients with multiple drug intolerances/failures. Yager et al. describe a successful case of a 69-year-old woman, where phenytoin was used to chemically cardiovert polymorphic ventricular tachycardia [1]. Phenytoin is a class 1B antiarrhythmic (similar to lidocaine and mexiletine) and is able to exert its antiarrhythmic properties through effects on both sodium and calcium channels in cardiac myocytes and purkinje cell membranes. It is important to note that, given its classification as a Vaughn William's class 1B antiarrhythmic it has weak affinity for the sodium channel and therefore weak sodium channel blockade in comparison to both class 1A and 1C antiarrhythmics which have moderate and strong sodium channel blockade, respectively. Phenytoin is able to effectively reduce the effective refractory period (ERP) on the cardiac conduction cycle unlike class 1A and 1C antiarrhythmics which increase or have no effect on the ERP, respectively. Although it is a weak sodium channel blocker in comparison to other class 1 antiarrhythmics, phenytoin finds its unique utility in terminating polymorphic ventricular tachycardia secondary to QT prolongation and should be considered in patients refractory to first line treatment modalities.

Phenytoin also has potential important toxicologic implications in the treatment of massive digoxin overdose. Rumack et al. describe a case of a

17-year-old patient with attempted suicide with a massive digoxin overdose successfully treated with phenytoin [2]. In overdose, digoxin can potentially precipitate fatal and life-threatening dysrhythmias, and phenytoin (and/or lidocaine) as class 1B antiarrhythmics are useful to suppress digitalis-induced tachydysrhythmias. Although not listed as an FDA approved indication, phenytoin and/or lidocaine should be considered in massive digoxin overdose as phenytoin is useful in suppressing the increased ventricular automaticity without suppressing atrial-ventricular (AV) conduction (enhances AV conduction) in the digitalis toxic patient. Phenytoin has been considered particularly useful because it does not decrease the inotropic effects of digitalis (which would be beneficial in a digoxin toxic patient), but rather suppresses supraventricular dysrhythmias [3]. Conclusively, phenytoin and/or lidocaine should be considered in digoxin-toxic patients who fail traditional therapy (e.g., Digifab, atropine, cardioversion, pacing, etc.) to suppress digitalis-induced tachydysrhythmias.

## DOSING (ADULT)

### Status Epilepticus (IV)

Neurocritical Care Society Recommendation:

- Loading dose: 20 mg/kg at a maximum rate of 50 mg/minute; if necessary, may give an additional dose of 5 to 10 mg/kg 10 minutes after the loading dose [4].

Manufacturer Recommendation:

- Loading dose: 10 to 15 mg/kg at a maximum rate of 50 mg/minute
- Initial maintenance dose (IV or oral): 100mg every 6 to 8 hours.

## Seizures (Non-Emergent)

*Oral*

Immediate release tablet:

- Initial: 100 mg 3 times daily, individualize dosage with dosage adjustments at no less than 7- to 10-day intervals.
- Maintenance dose: 300 to 400 mg/day; an increase to 600 mg/day may be necessary.

Immediate release Suspension:

- Initial: 125 mg 3 times daily, individualize dosage with dosage adjustments at no less than 7- to 10-day intervals; an increase to 625 mg/day may be necessary.

Extended release tablet:

- Loading dose: 1,000 mg divided into 3 doses (400, 300, 300 mg) administered at 2-hour intervals; begin maintenance dosage 24 hours after loading dose.

Note: Do not use loading dose regimen in patients with a history of renal or hepatic disease. Reserve for patients who require rapid steady state serum levels, when IV administration is not desirable, and for patients in a clinic or hospital setting where phenytoin levels can be closely monitored.

- Initial dosage (treatment naïve): 100 mg 3 times daily; adjust dosage at no less than 7- to 10-day intervals.
- Maintenance dose: 100 mg 3 to 4 times daily, doses up to 200 mg 3 times a day may be necessary. May consider converting patients established on 100 mg 3 times daily to 300 mg once daily.

## Dosing (Adult): Renal Impairment

There are no dosage adjustments provided in the manufacturer's labeling; <5% excreted as unchanged drug. Serum concentration may be difficult to interpret in renal failure. Monitoring of free (unbound) concentrations or adjustment to allow interpretation is recommended.

Hemodialysis: Dose supplementation may be required with high-efficiency dialyzers; monitor serum concentrations. Serum concentration may be difficult to interpret in renal failure [5-7].

## Dosing (Adult): Hepatic Impairment

There are no dosage adjustments provided in the manufacturer's labeling; undergoes hepatic metabolism and clearance may be decreased. Monitor free phenytoin levels closely. Dosage adjustments may be necessary.

## Dosing (Adult): Obesity

Evidence from one small study in adult patients (N = 24) with obesity (range: 71 to 197 kg) demonstrated that the volume of distribution ($V_d$) was 0.68 ± 0.03 L/kg (range: 0.53 to 0.85 L/kg) and distribution into weight in excess of IBW is disproportionately greater (by a factor of 1.33) [8].

## Loading Dose (Based on the Aforementioned Evidence)

- 14 mg/kg ideal body weight (IBW) + 19 mg/kg (weight in excess of IBW); maximum dose: 2,000 mg [8, 9].
- For example: For a patient with a total body weight (TBW) of 136 kg (300 lb.) and an IBW of 73 kg
- Loading dose = 14 mg/kg (73kg) + 19 mg/kg (136 kg minus 73 kg) = 2219 mg; administer the maximum dose of 2,000 mg.

## Alternative Strategy Targeting Specific Concentration

- May also target a specific concentration (e.g., 15 to 20 mg/L) by using the $V_d$ obtained from patients with obesity.[8, 10] Therefore, the concentration desired (in mg/L) may be multiplied by this $V_d$ (obesity) (in L) which is determined using the patient's total and ideal body weights.
- $V_d$ (obesity) = 0.65 L/kg [(IBW) + 1.33 (TBW – IBW)]
- Loading dose = calculated $V_d$ (obesity) (target concentration)
- For example: For a patient with a total body weight (TBW) of 136 kg (300 lb.) and an IBW of 73 kg
- $V_d$ (obesity) = 0.65 L/kg [(73kg) + 1.33 (136 kg – 73 kg)] = 101.9 L; then,
- Loading =101.9 L x 15 mg/L = 1,529 mg.

## Maintenance Dose

Base on IBW if using weight-based regimens or use conventional daily doses with adjustments based upon therapeutic drug monitoring and clinical effectiveness [8, 11].

Note: Additional data are necessary to further define dosing strategies in the obese patient. The above recommendations are based on a small study with a small sample size.

# ADMINISTRATION

## Vesicant/Purple Glove Syndrome (PGS)

*Introduction*

A thorough understanding of the importance of vesicants and the mechanism by which vesicants precipitate tissue necrosis is important as it pertains to phenytoin. The National Cancer Institute defines a vesicant as a drug that causes tissue injury after leaking out of a vein into the surrounding tissue (extravasation). Vesicants can cause severe blistering and other tissue injury that may be severe enough to lead to tissue necrosis (tissue death), ultimately requiring fasciotomies, amputations, and permanent disuse of the affected distal extremity [12, 13]. In addition to its other serious adverse effects (i.e., dermatologic reactions ranging from rashes to Stevens-Johnson syndrome or toxic epidermal necrolysis, and other hypersensitivity reactions), extravasation with associated soft tissue injury following IV phenytoin administration has been described numerous times in the literature dating back to the 1950s. In 1992, Hanna et al. described a delayed case of soft tissue injury of the hand and forearm following IV phenytoin administration and named it "purple glove syndrome (PGS)," owing to its unique purple phenotypic appearance [12]. Multiple reports began to surface following these initial reports, and it wasn't until November of 2011 that local toxicity information including PGS information was added to Pfizer's phenytoin (Dilantin) label. The revised label read as follows: "Soft tissue irritation and inflammation has occurred at the site of injection with and without extravasation of intravenous phenytoin. Edema, discoloration, and pain distal to the site of injection (described as "purple glove syndrome") have also been reported following peripheral intravenous phenytoin injection. Soft tissue irritation may vary from slight tenderness to extensive necrosis, and resolution of symptoms may be spontaneous, skin necrosis and limb ischemia have occurred and required such interventions such as fasciotomies, skin grafting, and, in rare cases, amputation."

## Mechanism of Vesicant/PGS

It is important to note that PGS can occur irrespective of the success of the IV catheter insertion as multiple cases have been reported after appropriate IV-line patency (adequate blood draw back, no inhibition of flow) with precipitation of the insidious onset of PGS [14]. The mechanism surrounding PGS associated with IV phenytoin administration has not been fully elucidated and is at best, speculative. Multiple theories have been proposed however a combination of theories seems more plausible given its complicated physiology. Many reports have proposed that the combination of small vascular tearing or micro-extravasation at the site of IV catheter insertion allow for leakage of phenytoin IV solution into surrounding tissue [15-17]. Phenytoin is commercially available as IV injection solution that is pH adjusted to a pH 12 with sodium hydroxide (NaOH) making this IV solution for injection extremely alkaline. This severe alkalinity can irritate the extravascular tissue (upon extravasation) causing soft tissue necrosis, disruption of endothelial barriers, and vasoconstriction [15-17]. Although this seems to be the predominant theory surrounding the mechanism of PGS, another theory postulates that the unique alkalinity of the IV phenytoin, once in contact with blood, leads to precipitation of certain compounds, leading to catheter obstruction and subsequent solution extravasation [17-19].

## Fosphenytoin (Cerebyx®) Reduced Potential for Extravasation/PGS

Fosphenytoin (Cerebyx®, Pfizer Inc., NY, NY), approved by the FDA in 1966, was marketed as the water-soluble prodrug of phenytoin. Following IV administration of fosphenytoin, it gets rapidly converted by phosphatases to the active drug of phenytoin to exert its therapeutic effect. Use of a water-soluble prodrug allowed for more rapid intravenous administration (three times as fast as phenytoin), averts the need for an intravenous filter, and allows for a lower potential for local tissue necrosis/soft tissue damage and cardiac toxicity. It is important to keep it mind that albeit reports of an improved safety profile, PGS has also been reported with IV fosphenytoin administration, although at a lower estimated incidence [20, 21].

## Treatment/Prevention of Extravasation/PGS

Caution is advised when administering phenytoin solution for injection due to its inherent basic pH: 12 (undiluted) making phenytoin IV solution a vesicant. Due to phenytoin's injectable solution high pH, subcutaneous (SubQ) administration is not recommended because of the possibility of local tissue damage. As mentioned previously, phenytoin is considered a vesicant, and therefore, when administered via the intravenous (IV) route and it is imperative to ensure proper needle or catheter placement prior to and during IV infusion to avoid extravasation. If extravasation occurs, stop the infusion immediately and disconnect (leave needle/cannula in place); gently aspirate extravasated solution (do NOT flush the line); remove needle/cannula and elevate extremity and apply to dry heat to promote lymphatic drainage. Closely monitor the patient for tissue sloughing or compartment syndrome as previous case reports of inadvertent compartment syndrome have been documented in the literature following phenytoin intravenous administration [22]. There is conflicting literature regarding treatment modalities (antidotal therapy) for extravasation management. Some sources recommend not to use an antidote with supportive care being sufficient [23] or to use hyaluronidase in refractory cases, [22] while other sources recommend hyaluronidase. Extravasation treatments for cytotoxic medications or vesicants such as that of phenytoin are centered around preventing additional tissue necrosis through inhibition of the drug spreading through additional extravascular tissue. Standard treatment consists of cessation of infusion and removing the cannula while elevating the limb to promote lymphatic drainage. If additional treatments are required based on the severity of extravasation, local irrigation using hyaluronidase and saline 0.9% can be considered to prevent further tissue necrosis. The literature surrounding the proposed mechanism for hyaluronidase is sparse and anecdotal however a few theories have been proposed. Hyaluronidase has been suggested to act via temporary breakdown of hyaluronic acid, which holds together tissue planes, and subsequent facilitation of drug dispersement and dilution [24]. The more concentrated the drug is in a particular area extravascularly is directly correlated with necrotic potential of that specific soft tissue. In cases of suspected PGS, limb angiography is often recommended for patients with signs and symptoms of altered perfusion of the affected extremity, consistent with potential PGS. Once vascular compromise is suspected and identification of ischemic progression of the suspected limb extremity is noted, consultation with vascular surgery is recommended to provide expert opinion. Both non-pharmacologic and pharmacologic treatment modalities are recommended however there is a paucity of data surrounding both of these potential treatment options. Hyaluronidase, IV steroids (hydrocortisone or triamcinolone), or heparin can be considered as previous case reports have purported their success and in the absence of contraindications should be considered [25-30]. It is worth reiterating that these treatment recommendations are experimental at best however immediate recognition and initiation of treatment is important to prevent irreversible ischemic changes that may lead to more extreme measures (i.e., fasciotomies or amputation).

## Risk of PGS in Non-Parenteral (Oral) Dosage Forms of Phenytoin

PGS associated with non-parenteral formulations is extremely rare, however two case reports have been reported in the literature following oral phenytoin administration. Yoshikawa et al. report the first case of a 10-year-old boy who was inadvertently administered an overdose of oral phenytoin suspension at a dose of 55mg/kg/day for 4 days instead of his prescribed 5.5 mg/kg/day (a 10-fold increase in his dose). The classic purple discoloration of his distal extremities developed several hours after his first toxic dose and disappeared 11 days after the drug was discontinued. The authors concluded that the development of PGS in this patient was multifactorial. A combination of the supratherapeutic plasma levels of phenytoin and the patient's significant comorbidities (spastic quadriplegia, severe mental retardation (MR), and epilepsy) jointly played a role in causing bilateral PGS in this patient's distal upper extremities [31]. 16 years later, a second case resurfaced regarding a 35-year-old man presenting with status epilepticus treated appropriately with phenytoin at an appropriate oral maintenance therapeutic dose following a loading dose of IV phenytoin ran at a rate of 20mg/min. 20 days following oral maintenance therapy (dose: 300mg/day), the patient reportedly developed bilateral pain and purple discoloration of his distal upper extremities. Symptomatology resolved following cessation of phenytoin therapy and replacement with oral valproic acid (VPA). The authors postulated the initial IV formulation was more of the causative agent inducing vasoconstriction and micro-thrombi formation [32]. As was the case for the initial patient case, chronic illness cannot be ruled out as a contributing risk factor and should always be taken into consideration; many of the times the diagnosis of PGS is a diagnosis of exclusion in the absence of any other precipitating factors/events. Given these two reports, albeit being extremely rare, monitoring for PGS during oral phenytoin (or any formulation for that matter), is warranted and providers should have a low index of suspicion should the patient develop any signs and symptoms consistent with PGS as mentioned in the previous section of this chapter.

## Summary/Recommendations

Local cutaneous reactions ranging from mild to severe are common during intravenous administration with both phenytoin and fosphenytoin (albeit at a much lower incidence due to its water-solubility). Severe forms of soft tissue injury, categorized as PGS, manifest as progressive skin discoloration (purple in phenotypic appearance), edema and pain at the site of extremity. If left untreated, symptomatology can progress to blistering, necrosis, or compartment syndrome. Should PGS continue to progress beyond these manifestations, interventions such as fasciotomies or skin grafts may be necessary to salvage remaining tissue or in cases with irreversible ischemic damage, amputation may be required.

Phenytoin and more recently, fosphenytoin, still remains the standard of care in the treatment of many seizures ranging from non-emergent seizures to status epilepticus despite local cutaneous reaction warnings put forth by the FDA. Should phenytoin and fosphenytoin be initiated in a patient where the clinician deems phenytoin a potential pharmacological agent, safety measures should be implemented to prevent the aforementioned local cutaneous reactions. First, large peripheral and central veins are recommended (preferably ultra-sound guided IVs if resources permit at a local institutional level), while avoiding small peripheral veins in the hand, wrist, or antecubital fossa. Second, meticulous adherence to recommended IV administration guidelines should be followed which include, appropriate dilution factors, correct administration rates, proper IV fluid choice, etc. Lastly, monitoring of the infusion site following IV infusion should be continuous to identify any early signs and symptoms that may be consistent with PGS or extravasation, especially in those patients unable to verbalize pain for whatever reason(s) (e.g., intubation, chronic illness precluding speech, etc.).

In the event of cutaneous soft tissue injury that is seen following phenytoin or fosphenytoin administration, appropriate measures should be taken to avoid morbidity and mortality. Immediate discontinuation of the offending agent along with frequent neurovascular assessments should be implemented to identify the extent (if any) of ischemic progression and to prevent subsequent tissue compromise; salvage measures should always be first priority. Angiography of the suspected limb or limbs is recommended if there is clinical suspicion for altered perfusion. Once vascular compromise is confirmed or suspected via angiography, involvement of or consultation with vascular surgery is highly recommended.

## IV Administration

IV administration (bolus/loading or continuous infusion) is associated with untoward side effects (e.g., hypotension and bradycardia) and caution should be advised with appropriate measures taken prior to administration (e.g., defibrillation pads, cardiac monitor, hemodynamic monitoring, etc.). The hypotension and bradycardia associated with phenytoin administration is a direct extrapolation of its effects at the sodium receptor (blockade). As is the case of many of the antiarrhythmics, reducing the upstroke and therefore the slope of phase 0 through sodium channel blockade in the cardiac conduction cycle will reduce dysrhythmias through a direct reduction in depolarization rate. This reduction in depolarization rate through sodium channel blockade will have the untoward effect of hypotension and bradycardia. Given the severity of this cardiovascular (CV) risk, The FDA has issued a US boxed warning for this potential CV toxicity associated with rapid infusion. Fosphenytoin may be considered for loading doses in patients who are in status epilepticus, hemodynamically unstable, or develop hypotension/bradycardia with IV administration of phenytoin. The mechanism surrounding this reduced incidence of cardiovascular compromise (hypotension and bradycardia) is a direct extension of its water-soluble properties. Although phenytoin may be administered by direct IV injection, it is preferable that phenytoin be administered via infusion pump either undiluted or diluted in normal saline (0.9%) as an IV piggyback (IVPB) to prevent exceeding the maximum infusion rate. As advised in the aforementioned paragraph, continuous monitoring and treatment for extravasation is important. Administer directly into a large peripheral or central vein through a large-gauge catheter. Infusion must be completed within 4 hours after dilution in normal saline.

The maximum rate of IV administration is 50mg/minute to prevent untoward hemodynamic instability (e.g., hypotension and bradycardia). Although the risk of cardiovascular toxicity increases with infusion rates above the recommended infusion rate, these events have also been reported at or below the recommended infusion rate. Reduction in rate of administration or discontinuation of dosing may be needed. Of note, fosphenytoin can be infused three times faster at a rate of 150mg/minute. Highly sensitive patients (e.g., elderly patients, patients with preexisting cardiovascular conditions) should receive phenytoin at a reduced rate (e.g., 20mg/minute) as a precaution [33].

When using IV route for oral replacement, administer at a slow rate as either a loading dose or by intermittent infusion. An in-line 0.22 to 0.55-micron filter is recommended for IVPB solutions due to the potential for precipitation of the solution. Following IV administration, normal saline (NS) should be injected through the same needle or IV catheter to prevent irritation.

## Administration Oral

Recommendations for the immediate release capsules/tablets include: dividing daily dose into 2 to 3 doses per day; if the daily dosage cannot be divided equally take the larger dose before bedtime.

Chewable tablets: May chew thoroughly before swallowing or swallow whole.

Suspension: Shake well prior to use to ensure uniformity of drug. Measure and administer dose using a calibrated oral dosing syringe (or other accurate dose-measuring device). Absorption is impaired when phenytoin suspension is given concurrently to patients who are receiving continuous nasogastric feedings and precautions should be taken (e.g., separating administration intervals or dividing the daily dose of phenytoin and withholding the administration of nutritional supplements for 1 to 2 hours before and after each phenytoin dose. The manufacturer recommends not to administer concomitantly with an enteral feeding preparation.

## Medication Guides

An FDA-approved patient medication guide, which is available with the product information, must be dispensed with phenytoin (all dosage forms).

# Storage

The appropriate storage for phenytoin is contingent on its dosage form and each manufacturer recommends different storage conditions based on the dosage form. Capsules and tablets are recommended to be stored at 20°C to 25°C (68°F to 77°F). In order to maintain stability and to ensure no loss in potency, the manufacturers recommend protecting the capsules from light and protecting the capsules and tablets from moisture. For the oral suspension, storage at 20°C to 25°C (68°F to 77°F) is recommended as well as avoiding exposure to light. Avoidance of direct light is recommended as well for the oral suspension. The storage for the injectable solution is unique compared to the other dosage forms and precautions should be taken to ensure appropriate storage to ensure no loss in potency. In accordance with the manufacturer recommendations, phenytoin solution for injection should be stored at 15°C to 30°C (59°F to 86°F). Additional recommendations for the injectable solution advise using only clear solutions free of precipitate and haziness however slightly yellow solutions may be used. Precipitation may occur if solution is solution is refrigerated and may dissolve at room temperature. Appropriate discarding of any unused production should be in accordance with local/health system protocols and guidelines.

# Monitoring

## General

Monitoring for phenytoin is extensive and is done to ensure patient's dose remains in the therapeutic range. Recommended monitoring parameters include: complete blood count (CBC), liver function; vitamin D status (chronic use); suicidality (e.g., suicidal thoughts, depression, behavioral changes); plasma phenytoin concentrations (if available, free phenytoin concentrations should be obtained in patients with renal impairment and/or hypoalbuminemia; if free phenytoin concentrations are unavailable, the adjusted total concentration may be determined based upon equation in adult patients (Corrected phenytoin = measured phenytoin level / ((adjustment x albumin, g/dL) + 0.1); adjustment = 0.275; in patients with creatinine clearance <20mL/min, adjustment + 0.2). This equation is colloquially known as the "Sheiner-Tozer equation" and is used to correct serum phenytoin levels for patients in renal failure or hypoalbuminemia defined as an albumin ≤3.2 g/dL (32g/L). Trough concentrations are generally recommended for routine monitoring. The rationale for obtaining phenytoin is explained in detail in the following section.

## Phenytoin Serum Levels

Obtaining serum phenytoin levels is not routinely performed, however in certain patient populations (e.g., renal failure and/or hypoalbuminemia), and those patients with a concern for a toxic ingestion, serums levels have a high level of clinical utility and implications for guiding therapy. Phenytoin is highly protein bound (87.8% to 91.9%) [34] however it is important to remember that it is the free drug (not bound to albumin) is the active drug. Many laboratories typically only measure the total phenytoin level, which can be problematic as the total phenytoin level encompasses both bound and unbound drug. The bound drug in the serum does not correlate with central nervous system (CNS) concentrations rather the unbound drug does, explaining the unbound serum level (or free drug) utility as an appropriate pharmacodynamic marker of bioavailability. In order to account for the free drug portion of phenytoin in the serum many equations have been developed, however the previously mentioned, Sheiner-Tozer equation is most widely used. Although this equation is helpful in determining unbound serum concentration, there are limitations to this formula as this formula was only studied, and therefore subsequently derived, from patients who were otherwise healthy [35]. Further research has shown it to have less utility and be less accurate in critically ill patients with renal failure or hypoalbuminemia. The albumin binding coefficient noted in the formula was derived from a range of studies however the most compelling data was from a study done by Cheng et al. which showed a coefficient of 0.275 to be most predictive, hence its presence in the current equation [36]. As clinicians when treating patients with either chronic phenytoin or phenytoin toxic patients, caution should be advised in patients whose disease states result in a decrease in serum albumin concentration as these patients will most benefit from the corrected serum phenytoin formula. These patients include those with: burns, hepatic cirrhosis, nephrotic syndrome, pregnancy, cystic fibrosis, etc. In addition, disease states resulting in an apparent decrease in affinity of phenytoin for serum albumin include, renal failure, jaundice (severe), other drugs (displacers), hyperbilirubinemia (total bilirubin >15mg/dL), CrCl <25 mL/min (unbound fraction is increased two-to threefold in uremia). Despite its seemingly important clinical implications, it is important to note that none of the equations (including the Sheiner-Tozer equation) has been validated by a prospective trial, and whenever possibly, free phenytoin levels should be used to guide therapy. The recommended therapeutic ranges are listed below for reference:

- Total phenytoin: 10 to 20 mg/L (SI: 40 to 79 micromole/L) (children and adults), 8 to 15mg/L (SI: 32 to 59 micromole/L) (neonates)
- Concentrations of 5 to 10 mg/L (SI: 20 to 40 micromole/L) may be therapeutic for some patients but concentrations <5 mg/L (SI: <20 micromole/L) are not likely to be effective
- 50% of patients show decreased frequency of seizures at concentrations >10 mg/L (SI: >40 micromole/L)
- 86% of patients show decreased frequency of seizures at concentrations >15 mg/L (SI: >59 micromole/L)
- Add another anticonvulsant if satisfactory therapeutic response is not achieved with a phenytoin concentration of 20 mg/L (SI: 79 micromole/L)

- Free phenytoin: 1 to 2.5 mg/L (SI: 4 to 10 micromole/L)
- Total phenytoin:
- Toxic: >30 mg/L (SI: >119 micromole/L)
- Lethal: >100 mg/L (SI: >396 micromole/L).

## When to Draw Phenytoin Serum Levels

As mentioned in the previous section, routine monitoring of phenytoin is not always clinically indicated however special populations, or those patients whose levels may be sub-therapeutic as a result of non-adherence may benefit from therapeutic monitoring to ensure clinical effectiveness. Time of phenytoin serum sampling is contingent on the disease state being treated and the clinical condition of the patient. Trough concentrations are generally recommended for routine monitoring as clinically indicated. However, timing of sampling is not as critical in patients receiving the extended-release dosage form (oral tablet) because the slow absorption minimizes the fluctuations between peak and trough concentrations. In general, serum concentrations should be drawn after a loading dose and in those patients on chronic phenytoin therapy at 3 to 12 month intervals. See below regarding the pertinent timing of when phenytoin serum levels should be drawn.

## After a Loading Dose

First concentration: It is recommended to draw within 2 to 3 days of therapy initiation to ensure the patient's metabolism is not remarkably altered. Alternatively, if rapid therapeutic levels are needed, a level may be drawn 2 hours after completion of an IV loading dose [33] or 24 hours after administration of an oral loading dose [37] to aid in determining maintenance dose or need to reload.

Second concentration: Draw within 5 to 8 days of therapy initiation with subsequent doses of phenytoin adjusted accordingly.

## Chronic Therapy

If plasma concentrations have not changed over a 3-to 5-day period, monitoring interval may be increased to once weekly in the acute clinical setting. In stable patients requiring long term therapy, monitor levels at 3-to 12-month intervals.

## Adjustment of Serum Concentrations When Free (Unbound) Serum Levels Are Unavailable

Obtaining free unbound serum concentrations are ideal to determine active phenytoin concentrations in patients with hypoalbuminemia or renal failure, it may not always be possible or feasible. If free unbound phenytoin concentrations are unattainable, there are equations that can be used to correct for both renal failure and hypoalbuminemia. There are two formulas that have become widely accepted and differ slightly for patients with low serum albumin or those patients with renal failure defined as a creatinine clearance ≤10mL/min. See below for the formula and correction charts for each patient population (low serum albumin and renal failure, respectively).

**Table 2.1. Adjustment of serum concentration in adults with hypoalbuminemia [38]**

| | Patient's Serum Albumin (g/dL) | | | |
|---|---|---|---|---|
| | 3.5 | 3 | 2.5 | 2 |

| Measured Total Phenytoin Concentration in mg/L (micromole/L) | Adjusted Total Phenytoin Concentration mg/L* (micromole/L) | | | |
|---|---|---|---|---|
| 5 (20) | 6 (24) | 7 (28) | 8 (32) | 10 (40) |
| 10 (40) | 13 (51.5) | 14 (55) | 17 (67) | 20 (79) |
| 15 (59) | 19 (75) | 21 (83) | 25 (99) | 30 (119) |

*Adjusted concentration = measured total concentration / [(0.2 x albumin) + 0.1].

**Table 2.2. Adjustment of serum concentration in adults with renal failure (CrCl ≤ 10 mL/min) [38]**

| Measured Total Phenytoin Concentration in mg/L (micromole/L) | Patient's Serum Albumin (g/dL) | | | | |
|---|---|---|---|---|---|
| | 4 | 3.5 | 3 | 2.5 | 2 |
| | Adjusted Total Phenytoin Concentration mg/L* (micromole/L) | | | | |
| 5 (20) | 10 (40) | 11 (44) | 13 (51.5) | 14 (55) | 17 (67) |
| 10 (40) | 20 (79) | 22 (87) | 25 (99) | 29 (115) | 33 (131) |
| 15 (59) | 30 (119) | 33 (131) | 38 (150) | 43 (170) | 50 (198) |

*Adjusted concentration = measured total concentration / [(0.1 x albumin) + 0.1].

## Additional Monitoring with IV Use

Continuous cardiac monitoring (rate, rhythm, blood pressure), and observation during administration is recommended to prevent untoward cardiovascular toxicity. Hemodynamics (including blood pressure and heart rate) should be monitored every 15 minutes for 1 hour after administration [33].

## Switching Formulations

Phenytoin base (e.g., oral suspension, chewable tablets) contain ~8% more drug than phenytoin sodium (~92mg base is equivalent to 100mg of phenytoin sodium). Dosage adjustments and closer serum monitoring may be necessary which switching dosage forms to avoid toxicity.

## REFERENCES


[1] Yager, N., Wang, K., Keshwani, N., & Torosoff, M. (2015). Phenytoin as an effective treatment for polymorphic ventricular tachycardia due to QT prolongation in a patient with multiple drug intolerances. *BMJ case reports*, *2015*, bcr2015209521. doi: 10.1136/ bcr-2015-209521.

[2] Rumack BH, Wolfe RR, Gilfrich H. Phenytoin (diphenylhydantoin) treatment of massive digoxin overdose. *Br Heart J*. 1974;36(4):405–408. doi:10.1136/hrt.36.4.405.

[3] Easterling R, Tietze PE. Digitalis toxicity. *J Am Board Fam Pract.* 1989;2:49-54.

[4] Brophy GM, Bell R, Claassen J, et al. Neurocritical Care Society Status Epilepticus Guideline Writing Committee. Guidelines for the evaluation and management of status epilepticus. *Neurocrit Care*. 2012;17(1):3-23.

[5] Asconapé JJ. Use of antiepileptic drugs in hepatic and renal disease. *Handb Clin Neurol*. 2014;119:417-432.

[6] Diaz A, Deliz B, Benbadis SR. The use of newer antiepileptic drugs in patients with renal failure. *Expert Rev Neurother*. 2012;12(1):99-105.

[7] Israni RK, Kasbekar N, Haynes K, Berns JS. Use of antiepileptic drugs in patients with kidney disease. *Semin Dial*. 2006;19(5):408-416.

[8] Abernethy DR and Greenblatt DJ, "Phenytoin Disposition in Obesity. Determination of Loading Dose," *Arch Neurol*, 1985;42(5):468-471.

[9] Erstad BL, "Dosing of Medications in Morbidly Obese Patients in the Intensive Care Unit Setting," *Intensive Care Med*, 2004, 30(1):18-32.

[10] Burton ME, Shaw LM, Schentag JJ, Evans WE. *Applied Pharmacokinetics and Pharmacodynamics*. Fourth ed. Baltimore, MD: Lippincott Williams & Wilkins; 2006.

[11] Erstad BL, "Which Weight for Weight-Based Dosage Regimens in Obese Patients?" *Am J Health-Syst Pharm*, 2002, 59:(21)2105-10.

[12] Hanna DR. Purple glove syndrome: A complication of intravenous phenytoin. *J Neurosci Nurs*. 1992;24(6): 340–345.

[13] Chokshi R, Openshaw J, Mehta NN, Mohler E., 3rd Purple glove syndrome following intravenous phenytoin administration. *Vasc Med.* 2007;12(1):29–31.

[14] Comer J. Extravasation from intravenous phenytoin. *Am J Intraven Ther Clin Nutr*. 1984;11:23–9.

[15] O'Brien T, Cascino G, So E, Hanna D. Incidence and clinical consequence of the purple glove syndrome in patients receiving intravenous phenytoin. *Neurology.* 1998;51(4):1034–9. doi: 10.1212/WNL.51.4.1034.

[16] Spengler R, Arrowsmith J, Kilarski D, Buchanan C, Von Behren L, Graham D. Severe soft-tissue injury following intravenous infusion of phenytoin. Patient and drug administration risk factors. *Arch Intern Med.* 1988; 148(6):1329–33. doi: 10.1001/archinte.1988.00380060093019.

[17] Jamerson B, Dukes G, Brouwer K, Donn K, Messenheimer J, Powell J. Venous irritation related to intravenous administration of phenytoin versus fosphenytoin. *Pharmacother: J Hum Pharmacol Drug Ther.* 1994;14(1):47–52.

[18] Doellman D, Hadaway L, Bowe-Geddes L, Franklin M, LeDonne J, Parke-O'Donnell L, et al. Infiltration and extravasation. Update on prevention and management. *J Infus Nurs*. 2009;32(4):203–11. doi: 10.1097/NAN.0b013e3181aac042.

[19] Hannon M, Lee S. Extravasation injuries. *J Hand Surg.* 2011;36A:2060–5. doi: 10.1016/j.jhsa.2011.10.001.

[20] *Cerebyx (Fosphenytoin Sodium Injection) (prescribing information).* Pfizer Labs: New York. Revised April 2014. http://labeling.pfizer.com/ShowLabeling.aspx?id=749. Accessed 11 July 2019.

[21] *Intravenous Phenytoin and Fosphenytoin Safety Concerns Background Package*. Available at: http://www.fda.gov/downloads/advisorycommittees/committeesmeetingmaterials/drugs/peripheralan

dcentralnervoussystemdrugsadvisorycommittee/ucm231776.pdf. Accessed 11 July 2019.

[22] Reynolds PM, MacLaren R, Mueller SW, Fish DN, Kiser TH. Management of extravasation injuries: a focused evaluation of noncytotoxic medications. *Pharmacotherapy*. 2014;34(6):617-632. doi: 10.1002/phar.1396.

[23] Montgomery LA, Hanrahan K, Kottman K, et al. Guideline for I.V. infiltrations in pediatric patients. *Pediatr Nurs*. 1999;25(2):167-169, 173-180.

[24] Marders J. Sounding the alarm for I.V. infiltration. *Nursing*. 2005; 35(4):18–20. doi: 10.1097/00152193-200504000-00012.

[25] Prasad R, Mishra O, Gupta A. Gangrene of left hand following accidental intra-arterial injection of phenytoin sodium. *Pediatric Oncall* (serial online) 2012. doi: 10.7199/ped.oncall.2012.28.

[26] Sintenie J, Tuinebreijer W, Kreis R, Breederveld R. Digital gangrene after accidental intra-arterial injection of phenytoin (Epanutin) *Eur J Surg*. 1992;158(5):315–6.

[27] Mahajan R, Batra Y, Rajeev S. Intravenous phenytoin and percutaneous arterial cannulation: the purple-glove syndrome. *Eur J Anaesthesiol.* 2007; 24(10):900–1. doi: 10.1017/S0265021507001 007.

[28] Scumpia A, Yahsou J, Cajina J, Cao C. Purple glove syndrome after intravenous phenytoin administration presenting in the emergency department. *J Emerg Med*. 2013; 44(2):e281–3. doi: 10.1016/j. jemermed.2012.07.057.

[29] McLean C, Cheng K, Clifton M. Fatal case of accidental intra-arterial phenytoin injection. *Eur J Vasc Endovasc Surg*. 2002;23(4):378–9. doi: 10.1053/ejvs.2001.1586.

[30] Keane M, Shirazi H, Marsh P, Khushal A. Purple glove syndrome following intravenous phenytoin infusion. *Br J Surg*. 2009; 96(9): 1065.

[31] Yoshikawa H, Abe T, Oda Y. Purple glove syndrome caused by oral administration of phenytoin. *J Child Neurol*. 2000;15(11):762. doi: 10.1177/088307380001501110.

[32] Jain RS, Nagpal K, Kumar S, Prakash S, Handa R. Purple glove syndrome occurring after oral administration of phenytoin in therapeutic doses: mechanism still a dilemma. *Am J Emerg Med.* 2015;33(1):123.e5–123.e6. doi: 10.1016/j.ajem.2014.05.039.

[33] Meek PD, Davis SN, Collins DM, et al. "Guidelines for Nonemergency Use of Parenteral Phenytoin Products: Proceedings of an Expert Panel Consensus Process. Panel on Nonemergency Use of Parenteral Phenytoin Products," *Arch Intern Med*, 1999, 159(22): 2639-44.

[34] Richens A. Clinical pharmacokinetics of phenytoin. *Clin Pharmacokinet*. 1979; 4(3):153-169.

[35] Martin E, Tozer TN, Sheiner LB, Reigelman S. The Clinical Pharmacokinetics of phenytoin. *J Pharmacokinet Biopharm.* 1977 Dec;5(6):579-96.

[36] Cheng W, Kiang TKL, Bring P, Ensom MHH. Predictive Performance of the Winter-Tozer and Derivative Equations for Estimating Free Phenytoin Concentration. *The Canadian Journal of Hospital Pharmacy*. 2016;69(4):269-279.

[37] Osborn HH, Zisfein J, Sparano R. Single-dose oral phenytoin loading. *Ann Emerg Med*. 1987;16(4):407-412.

[38] Phenytoin. *Lexi Drugs. Lexicomp*. Wolters Kluwer Health, Inc. Riverwoods, IL. Available at http://online.lexi.com. Accessed June 30th, 2019.

In: The Pharmacological Guide to Phenytoin ISBN: 978-1-53616-980-5
Editor: Payal Sud 

*Chapter 3*

# SPECIAL POPULATIONS

***Michael K. Connolly**, MD***
Hackettstown Emergency Medical Associates LLC,
Department of Emergency Medicine,
Hackettstown, NJ, US

## ABSTRACT

This chapter will consider selected populations that require special attention with regards to the administration of phenytoin. It is important for clinicians to be aware of the variables at play that make these populations unique in order for therapy to be tailored thus avoiding toxicity. The neonatal and pediatric populations will be the focus, with some remarks on patients with liver and/or kidney impairment. This chapter will focus primarily on the alterations of the pharmacokinetics in these populations since most of the susceptibility to toxicity are due to these differences. Differences in the pharmacokinetics of these populations as compared to the general population requires caution and special attention to dosing, drug level monitoring, focused history and examination, and the recognition/management of toxicity.

* Corresponding Author's Email: michaelkevinconnolly@gmail.com.

Preceding the highlights of special considerations in the neonatal and pediatric populations will be a discussion on phenytoin's historical and present role in the management of childhood epilepsy. Trends in phenytoin's use as compared to other traditional antiepileptic drugs (AEDs) will be discussed in the context of the available literature. Focus will turn to the general physiological and pharmacological differences between the neonatal/pediatric populations as compared to the general population. This will highlight important principles necessary to understand how some of these differences pertain specifically to the administration of phenytoin in these populations. Age dependent adverse effects will be explored with regards to differences in incidence and presentation in these populations. Finally, special consideration relating to the history, physical and management primarily pertaining to the evaluation of phenytoin toxicity will be considered.

A vast majority of medications are affected by alterations in hepatic and renal function. Phenytoin is a classic example of how impairments in either the liver or kidneys can dramatically alter phenytoin concentrations predisposing these populations at increased risk for toxicity.

Unfortunately, evidence-based research is often scarce and limited in these special populations. This is not only true of phenytoin but a common limitation in the evaluation and understanding of many medications that are commonly used in these populations. Very few randomized trials are available in support of the information contained in this chapter. Rather, literature will often be dependent on available observational and case reports/series studies. While limitations in available literature is common, this chapter will provide information valuable to the health care provider in order to make cognizant decisions and recommendations to patients in these special populations.

## INTRODUCTION

Phenytoin was discovered in 1908 and for over half a century has been one of the most studied and administered anticonvulsants in all populations for the management of acute seizures and epilepsy [1, 2]. Seizures have a prevalence of 0.5-1% in the general population and are among the most common chronic neurological disorders in the neonatal and pediatric populations [3]. Childhood diagnosed epilepsy has an estimated incidence of 41-187/100,000 with an annual diagnosis of about 30,000 children and adolescents [3, 4]. Specific to the neonatal population, seizures from any cause are estimated to account for 2-4 per 1000 North American births with 19-58 per 1000 in birth weight infants [5-8]. Preterm neonates are at an especially increased risk for the development of seizures and are also more likely to develop significant morbidity and mortality [5]. In one prospective study carried out in a neonatal unit of a tertiary hospital, morbidity and mortality was associated with prematurity, low birth weight, low Apgar score at 5 minutes, meningitis, sepsis, severe hypoxic-ischemic encephalopathy (HIE), brain malformations, grade 3 or 4 intraventricular or intracranial hemorrhage, seizure onset <24 hours, presence of status epilepticus, and severely abnormal radiological and EEG findings [5]. Sepsis and HIE were found to be associated with the greatest risk which has also been cited in prior studies [5, 9].

Long-term anticonvulsant therapy is the mainstay of treatment for epilepsy, in addition to its use as adjunctive therapy to first line benzodiazepines in the management of status epilepticus. In current practice, seizure prophylaxis for the management of cerebral vascular accidents has seen a decline in use due to questionable effectiveness in changing outcomes and even potentially worsening outcomes. In general, AEDs have significantly grown over the past 20 years and are commonly classified as 1st, 2nd or 3rd generation AEDs. [Table 3.1] Despite the increased growth of newer AEDs over the past few decades, traditional AEDs (1st generation), such as phenytoin and phenobarbital, still remain popular drugs for the management of seizure disorders in the neonatal/pediatric populations as well as the general population [1, 5, 10]. Popularity of phenytoin is not limited to the U.S. but a common AED world-wide. In fact, the World Health Organization (WHO) lists phenytoin on their List of Essential Medicines [2]. Phenytoin and fosphenytoin, a water soluble phosphorylated pro-drug of phenytoin, are not without their limitations despite ongoing popularity in both the neonatal and pediatric populations. Both have a relatively narrow therapeutic index as compared to other anticonvulsants especially newer 2nd and 3rd generation AEDs [2]. However, familiarity and the lack of strong evidence supporting the superiority of other AEDs in managing neonatal and pediatric seizure disorders are likely reasons for their continued popularity.

It is important to note, that although there has been no strong evidence favoring the effectiveness of newer anticonvulsants over phenytoin, the available literature is limited in this regard. This especially holds true in both the neonatal and pediatric populations. In particular, most drug dosing in neonates are extrapolated from older children and the adult populations [11, 12]. Despite the expansion in neonatal anticonvulsant therapies over the past 20 years, phenytoin/fosphenytoin remains a popular choice among clinicians despite seizure control in less than half of neonates treated individually with either phenobarbital or phenytoin in one study [10]. This is in addition to specific concerns within this population in terms of less predictable pharmacology and the propensity for the development of toxicity given phenytoin/fosphenytoin's narrow therapeutic index, potential medication interactions, and need for frequent blood draws necessary for blood-level monitoring [5, 10]. Long-term management with oral phenytoin for the management of neonatal and pediatric epilepsy is also not without its potential for chronic toxicity which will be described later in this chapter as compared to the general population. As mentioned, the literature is limited primarily to case reports and studies on the effectiveness of phenytoin in both acute seizure management and long-term use for epilepsy.

## NEONATES AND PEDIATRIC POPULATION

### Neonates: Evidence Based Trends for the Use of Phenytoin in Seizure Disorders

A systematic review by Slaughter et al. evaluated the available literature in determining the most effective anticonvulsant therapy in neonatal seizures [5]. A total of 16 studies were included in the analysis and were subdivided into tiers based on the quality of research design. Tier 1 studies required studies with control or comparison groups and of the 16 studies, only 4 met this requirement for which 2 of these controlled studies were randomized. Of the two randomized studies, one evaluated phenytoin which was compared against phenobarbital [10, 13]. Tier 2 designation consisted of 11 studies but the design of many of these studies was limited by not having a control or comparison group. Painter et al. conducted the only randomized control study on phenytoin for the treatment of neonatal seizures in 1999. In this study, from 1990 to 1995, 59 neonates with seizures confirmed by electroencephalography (EEG) were randomized to either receive IV phenytoin with a free plasma concentration of 3 mg/L or phenobarbital with a free level achieved at 25 mg/L. Patients who failed initial therapy were crossed to receive both therapies. Seizures were controlled in 45% (13 of 29 neonates) of patients in the phenytoin group and 43% (13 of 30 neonates; P = 1) in the phenobarbital group. Analysis of cross over patients revealed ultimate seizure control in 62% vs 57%, respectively (P = 0.67). Therefore, while both groups were fairly equal in efficacy, overall the results show that any single agent is less than ideal. Interestingly, this study observed no adverse effects despite a somewhat concerning toxicological profile for both phenytoin and phenobarbital. Phenobarbital overdose can result in over-sedation risking aspiration and rhabdomyolysis in addition to respiratory failure which can lead to apnea-induced cardiac arrest and global hypoxic injury. As will be discussed in more detail later, phenytoin has a relatively low therapeutic range with the potential for toxicity with even mildly elevated supratherapeutic serum concentrations. This study also found poorer outcomes in patients with more severe presentations of their seizure independent of the agent(s) used to control them. This was highlighted by the fact that neonates with milder seizures prior to therapy tended to have termination of seizure activity regardless of the anticonvulsant used. Two limitations worth noting in this study were single center design possibly limiting external generalizability and single-blinding design, as both physicians and EEG technicians were aware of the treatment groups.

It is important to note, while phenobarbital and phenytoin have traditionally been popular anticonvulsants in both of these populations, newer generation AEDs (in particular levetiracetam) have gained popularity primarily due to safer toxicological profiles. However, no AEDs in a well-controlled study have shown superiority over phenobarbital or phenytoin [5]. One concern of phenytoin use in the neonatal population are the frequent blood draws in some circumstances risking anemia and morbidity from required blood transfusions [5]. Also, as will be discussed later in this chapter, neonatal pharmacokinetics (absorption, distribution, metabolism, and excretion) are often less predictable in this population with high degrees of variability. This places this particular population at an increased risk for phenytoin poisoning. When comparing phenytoin to phenobarbital, the former is significantly less likely to cause sedative-hypotonic related toxicity [1]. Therefore, clinicians should be aware of how older versus newer generation AEDs compare in terms of overall efficacy, adverse effect profile, dosing regimens, compliance, and any further considerations related to higher risk populations. While literature is limited in the neonatal and pediatric populations for phenytoin and other older traditional AEDs, even more so with newer generation AEDs that are currently available. It is possible that future studies will reveal superiority of these newer generation AEDs in terms of the above-mentioned parameters. Regardless, conventional AEDs are likely to remain popular choices for years to come.

Despite the lack of literature in support of newer AEDs in the neonatal population, some studies have shown a trend in prescribing practices favoring some newer generation agents [5, 14, 15]. Due to the questionable efficacy of older AEDs (including phenytoin), Silverstein and Ferriero [14] conducted a 2007 survey to determine trends in the prescribing patterns of pediatric neurologists for the management of neonatal seizures. This study was conducted within the context of reports from prior studies reporting higher frequency of these newer off-label agents despite lack of information supporting their efficacy and safety. Surveys were distributed to pediatric neurologists from multiple sites with 55 respondents. Specifically, 73% of respondents reported the use of either levetiracetam, topiramate, or both. Levetiracetam was used by 47% (26 of 55) of responders, while 55% (30 of 55) used topiramate. It was noted in this study that in the majority of cases, prescribers believed these medications to be efficacious.

In a more recent study on use of newer off-label agents, Ahmad et al. [15] conducted a retrospective cohort study on a large, deidentified multicenter data set to evaluate treatment trends in the ICU setting from 2005 to 2014. They hypothesized a growing trend in these newer agents, in particular levetiracetam. Similar to Silverstein and Ferriero's study, they observed a growing trend in the use of these newer agents and a decline in the use of more conventional antiepileptics. They identified 9134 neonates diagnosed with a seizure disorder and who received an antiepileptic medication during their stay in the NICU prior to discharge. Levetiracam exposure increased from 1.4 to 14% ($P < 0.001$), a ten-fold increase during this time period. Phenobarbital, while still popular, saw a decrease in use from 99% to 96% ($P < 0.001$) and phenytoin from 15 to 11% ($P < 0.001$). Off-label AEDs, such as carbamazepine and topiramate accounted for <1%. Therefore, this study revealed a significant decrease in the use of phenytoin with the replacement of levetiracetam as the second most common agent used and with phenobarbital remaining number one despite the small decrease in use. It is unclear exactly the reason for this decline especially with the lack of research in support of these newer agents, but likely personal clinical experiences revealing safer profiles while maintaining the same or greater efficacy, easier monitoring, and/or increased compliance are driving factors for this.

## Pediatrics: Evidence Based Trends for the Use of Phenytoin in Seizure Disorders

Similar to prescribers in the neonatal population, there are also concerns over the efficacy and safety of conventional AEDs in the management of seizure disorders in the pediatric population [16, 17]. Like the neonatal population, conventional AEDs had been the mainstay of treatment but with a growing trend of newer AEDs on the market, prescribing and administration patterns are changing. In particular, valproic acid (VPA) and carbamazepine (CBZ) have traditionally been popular agents in the pediatric population. Prior to the late 2000's, VPA was the most common AED; however, recent trends have seen a decrease in VPA use and an increase in the use of newer 2$^{nd}$ and 3$^{rd}$ generation AEDs [16]. In a cross-sectional study by Liu et al. [16] trends in AED use in children and adolescence were evaluated. Data was reviewed from 26 US states via the Medicaid Analytic eXtract data set. A patient was defined as age 3 to 18 with at least a one-day supply of the AED during the 1-year follow-up period. They evaluated 11 cohorts which ranged between 17,304 and 22,672 patents and found the following prevalence trends between 1999 to 2009: (1) VPA: declined from 42.4% to 26.5; (2) CBZ: declined from 37.1% to 10.2%; (3) Levetiracetam: increased from 5.1% to 32.0%; and (4) Oxcarbazepine: increased from 1.3% to 19.1%. Towards the end of the study period in 2008, levetiracetam surpassed VPA in popularity. The authors noted fewer adverse effects and increased adherence as the main factors for this trend. However, similar to the neonatal population, evidence for safety and cost effectiveness is lacking. Research on AED in both the neonatal and pediatric population has traditionally been limited and information often derived from adult studies. Insufficient population size, short duration of treatments, and/or lack of controlled studies are some reasons for this [17].

In summary, the neonatal and pediatric populations have some differences. With the neonatal population, over the past 20 years, phenytoin use has decreased and levetiracetam has increased; however, phenobarbital has remained fairly steady. While phenytoin has decreased it still remains a popular choice. In the pediatric population, a similar trend with the increase use of levetiracetam has been observed. While the older conventional AED VPA remains a popular choice in the pediatric population, it too has seen a dramatic decrease in use over the last 2 decades. Phenytoin is significantly less prescribed in the pediatric population as compared to the neonatal population overall. With newer and likely safer agents, phenytoin will likely continue to trend down in overall use. Regardless, clinicians should be cognizant of the cons of phenytoin. As mentioned above, its narrower therapeutic index and less predictable pharmacokinetic profile are the main concerns which will be described in greater detail later in this chapter.

**Table 3.1. Classification of Antiepileptic Medications by Generation**

| 1st Generation | 2nd Generation | 3rd Generation |
|---|---|---|
| Carbamazepine | Felbamate | Brivaracetam |
| Clonazepam | Gabapentin | Eslicarbazepine |

| | | |
|---|---|---|
| Ethosuximide<br>Phenobarbital<br>Phenytoin<br>Primidone<br>Valproic Acid | Lamotrignine<br>Levetiracetam<br>Oxcarbazepine<br>Pregabalin<br>Topiramate<br>Zonisamide | Ezogabine<br>Lacosamide<br>Perampanel<br>Rufinamide<br>Stiripentol |

In order to illustrate the differences within these populations as compared to the general population from a pharmacological standpoint, we will first explore basic pharmacological differences within both of these groups as compared the general population and later hone in on specific pharmacological issues that are seen with the use of phenytoin.

## Pharmacological Differences and Considerations Unique to the Neonatal and Pediatric Populations

Age-related differences in both pharmacokinetics and pharmacodynamics are critical to understand in order to appreciate the differences between populations based on age. From the newborn to the adolescent, maturity in certain physiological parameters often dictate response to certain medications. The differences account for therapeutic onset, bioavailability, metabolism to inactive and/or active metabolites, and elimination. One or more of these pharmacological parameters can tilt the desired therapeutic effect of medications to toxicity. The expression that children are not small adults highlights this principle. However, weight-based dosing is often extrapolated to children from adult data secondary to the not uncommon lack of pharmacokinetic/dynamic studies in these populations. This poses a significant risk for the development of toxicity and therefore the clinician should be cognizant of certain important pharmacological and physiological differences in these two populations in order to optimize therapy and decrease risk for toxicity. This especially holds true for phenytoin and other 1$^{st}$ generation AEDs which are collectively characterized by higher protein binding and significant drug to drug interactions which need to be accounted for. This next section will highlight some important differences and will be divided into the following phases: absorption, distribution, metabolism, and excretion. This will be followed by a more in-depth analysis of pharmacological differences in both the pediatric and neonatal populations with regards to phenytoin administration.

*Absorption*

Developmental changes within the absorptive surfaces of the gastrointestinal (GI) tract alter the absorption of certain medications and thus the bioavailability. Gastric pH is also another consideration when administering *per os* (PO) route medications. Gastric pH immediately after birth is near neutral which rapidly drops to a pH of 1-3 after 24 hours from birth. This drop is only transient as it rises again to near neutral by day 10 and again drops slowly to adult levels fully by roughly age 3 [19-21]. In pre-term infants, gastric pH is affected and may not follow this pattern but rather has minimal to no free gastric acid production [19, 21]. This can significantly decrease dissolution and absorption of certain medications depending on the dissolution environment required of some medications. For example, drugs such as phenytoin and phenobarbital are weak acids. The enteral formulation of phenytoin is up to 75% absorbed, a reduction from adult level of 100% absorption [19, 22]. Gastric emptying and intestinal motility is also age-dependent. In general, neonates and young infants tend to have slower gastric emptying and it would be expected that bioavailability would be increased in these age groups secondary to increased mucosal surface contact time; however, certain medications have shown to have delayed and incomplete absorption [19, 23]. Absorption is a dynamic process and many factors govern the ultimate passage from within the gastrointestinal tract into systemic circulation. For example, administration of fat-soluble xenobiotics may have decreased absorption during the first few months of life secondary to an immature and still developing GI exocrine system. Bile salt content and enterohepatic re-circulation of bile develops during this time and are both premature until months after birth [24, 25]. Absorption is also affected by the gastrointestinal bacterial milieu that starts to colonize infants within hours following birth. Intestinal flora is likely highly variable between age groups and even within the same age groups. For example, breastfed infants may have different flora as compared to formula fed infants [24, 26]. It is unclear what effect the variability in the intestinal flora between and within age groups has on the pharmacokinetics of drugs but likely has some level of impact on absorption and bioavailability of certain medications.

*Routes of Administration*

Bioavailability of a drug is dependent on the route of administration. Enteral administration may have varying degrees of rates between and within each age group for all the reasons explained above. However, on the other end of the spectrum, the intravenous (IV) route has 100% bioavailability as it is directly introduced into systemic circulation and is not dependent on the various pharmacological parameters that govern enteral, intramuscular (IM), intranasal (IN), dermal, subcutaneous (SQ), intrathecal/spinal, and rectal administration. Each of these routes have intrinsic factors at play governing bioavailability regardless of age. However, neonates and smaller children have unique physical and/or physiological differences that influence bioavailability regardless of the medication administered.

For example, the IM route is dependent on skeletal muscle volume, vascularity and perfusion of these muscles, and the administered volume [19]. During the first month of life, owing to reduced muscle mass and higher proportion of water per body surface area, administration via the IM route is less than ideal in the neonatal period. Medications administered via this route in the newborn period are absorbed erratically and with unpredictable pharmacokinetics and therefore reliance on other parenteral routes such as the SQ route are more reliable [19, 24, 27].

Transmucosal routes, such as the rectal route can be useful when patients are on PO restriction and/or unable to tolerate PO. The rectal route is not uncommonly utilized during hospitalization in all age groups. However, the rectal route is often limited by the manufacture of certain medications and/or unfavorable inherent chemical properties of either the medication and/or their vehicles for administration and absorption. Further, certain formularies may be irritating to the rectal mucosa as compared to other routes. Successful absorption via the rectal route is heavily dependent on regional vascularity. Unlike the IM route which is dependent on the still immature skeletal vascularity, the rectal vascular maturation process is near complete which sets up an ideal environment for adequate absorption [19]. Most of the variability seen between different age groups is secondary to the location of rectal medication administration. For example, lower rectal applications are systemically absorbed and bypass first pass metabolism. Medications deposited higher in the rectum get absorbed into the portal system and thus may undergo first pass hepatic metabolism. Therefore, neonatal and younger children who have immature CYP 450 metabolism may have a different bioavailability profile as compared to older children and adults [28]. The oral mucosal route (sublingual, buccal) can also be an ideal alternative in patients that are NPO. However, unlike the rectal route, smaller children are more likely to swallow significant quantities of the drug. This not only results in the utilization of favorable pharmacokinetics intrinsic to the mucosal route, such as, avoidance of gastric pH degradation and bypassing enterohepatic circulation, but can also result in more delayed absorption from the gut. Therefore, this route is less ideal in the pediatric population, especially smaller children who are unable to maintain adequate mucosal contact while increasing ingestion of the drug [28].

The percutaneous route via a patch delivery system or applied cream can be administered with great results in certain scenarios. Absorption is dependent on the thickness of the epidermal stratum corneum. Neonates and smaller infants have a thinner layer as compared to older children and adults. Therefore, the rate and extent of certain dermal preparations are often more rapidly absorbed. While this can be of great benefit, this also runs the risk for toxicity based on rate related reasons and increased bioavailability [19, 27, 28]. In addition to the unpredictable pharmacokinetics with transdermal delivery systems, iatrogenic or inadvertent dosing at home may occur when patches are applied without removing older ones.

*Distribution*

The distribution of the drug to various compartments is an especially important pharmacological phase that differs from adults. Distribution is primarily dependent on the solubility of a drug, and percentage of protein binding. More lipophilic drugs are able to cross into the plasma membranes of cells and distribute deep into various compartments. However, lipophilic drugs require protein binding while in the plasma and only the unbound fraction is readily available to distribute and be pharmacologically active.

Neonates often have less predictable protein binding and therefore distribution. In general, neonates as compared to adults and older children have less protein binding secondary to decreased affinity for the carrier protein and decreased quantity of protein carriers such as albumin. Newborns still have a fraction of fetal albumin which has less of an affinity for drug binding [29-32]. Albumin concentration nears adult levels at 12 months of life. Endogenous compounds such as bilirubin compete for albumin binding sites [29]. Decreased protein binding in neonates and younger infants results in increased distribution and can lend to potential toxicity. This also holds true for patients with conditions resulting in hypoalbuminemia, such as liver and renal disease. Drug penetration into the neonatal central nervous system is also increased as compared to the general population for a few reasons. Higher serum concentrations of lipophilic drugs secondary to decreased protein binding sets up a stronger concentration gradient at the blood brain barrier (BBB). Neonates also have a higher relative brain weight as well as a higher ratio of cerebral to systemic blood flow [29, 33]. Lastly, both the blood-brain and blood-CSF barriers are thought to be underdeveloped and immature lending to leaky cerebral vasculature and thus less control on drug penetration into the CNS [29-31, 34]. For all of the above reasons, neonates and young infants are at increased risk for toxicity by increased distribution to deeper compartments. Decreased protein binding and less restriction into the CNS account for the main distribution differences in this population as compared to the general population.

### *Metabolism and Elimination*

Metabolism of drugs can occur in a variety of places including the plasma and within tissues of just about any organ, with the liver being the most important. Metabolism in the liver is dependent on an array of enzymes, most important of which are the CYP450 class. This class may be either absent, deficient or functionally immature early in life and require time to mature. As such, neonates are prone to incomplete metabolism in a variety of xenobiotics that depend on this enzyme system [18]. In general, metabolism of drugs results in the production of inactive metabolites which intimately ties metabolism to elimination. However, some drugs produce active but less potent metabolites (e.g., diazepam), while others metabolize to more potent pharmacologically active compounds as compared to their parent compound (e.g., codeine). Finally, some medications are considered prodrugs which are pharmacologically inactive and require metabolism to produce the active form. An example of this is fosphenytoin which differs from phenytoin by a phosphate ester group and after being metabolized by plasma and tissue specific phosphatases, active phenytoin is released [35]. It is important for clinicians to be aware of basic metabolism which can have significant toxicological implications. For example, codeine is metabolized by CYP 2D6 into morphine and a small percentage of children were found to be rapid metabolizers resulting in increased concentrations of morphine resulting in significant morbidity and mortality [77].

Elimination of a drug is a dynamic process that starts once absorption begins. Some medications are eliminated without significant metabolism as parent compounds while others are first metabolized. Commonly, medications are metabolized and eliminated in certain percentages by more than one end organ. For example, biliary elimination and renal elimination can take place simultaneously in varying percentages. Renally excreted drugs can have variability in half-lives solely based on the processes that govern renal elimination, many of which require maturation after birth. Renal elimination matures with gestational age and body weight [35]. Renal elimination is dependent on simultaneous mechanisms such as glomerular filtration, tubular secretion and reabsorption [29]. Glomerular Filtration Rate (GFR) is lowest in neonates as compared with children and adults. GFR rapidly increases during the first two weeks of life and eventually reaches adult rates at 6-12 months. Preterm infants have a similar pattern although time to reach adult levels is delayed making this population especially susceptible to medications that are renally eliminated [29, 34-36]. Tubular secretion and reabsorption are also immature at birth and are approximately

25% of adult values [29, 34]. While active tubular secretion mechanisms mature within the same time frame as glomerular filtration, tubular reabsorption is a gradual process which reaches adult levels during adolescence [29].

## Pharmacological Considerations Specific to Phenytoin in the Neonatal and Pediatric Age Groups

Now that this chapter has highlighted some important age-related pharmacological differences, a more focused discussion on how these differences pertain to the administration of phenytoin will follow. This section will first hone in on the most clinically relevant factors that clinicians should be aware of followed by some further considerations that may lack clear clinical relevance secondary to limited research, conflicting evidence, or a reliance on anecdotal information. Therefore, it is important to understand that some of these pharmacological considerations have unclear relevance to clinical practice, in part due to the lack of available age specific pharmacokinetic and pharmacodynamic studies at present.

Phenytoin is primarily administered orally or intravenously and fosphenytoin is only intravenously administered. This is true for all populations. The IM route is not recommended secondary to poor solubility and thus erratic absorption. As mentioned above, the IM route within itself is not an ideal route of administration for most medications in the neonatal and pediatric populations secondary to decreased muscle mass and vascularity. Absorption after oral administration can potentially vary among age groups based on gastric pH differences. Since phenytoin is a weak acid, the enteral formulation may have some degree of incomplete absorption when compared to adults. This may be more significant for pre-term neonates where gastric acid output may be minimal. Neonates and infants up to 4 months of age can have an approximately 75% decrease in absorption as compared to complete absorption in adults [22]. One significant consideration of the intravenous route in these younger populations is the risk for extravasation. Risk of extravasation is increased in the pediatric population secondary to the small diameter of veins and therefore special attention is warranted to ensure that access is sufficient prior to administering phenytoin or fosphenytoin. Fosphenytoin is more water soluble and thus less likely to cause significant complications after extravasation but necrosis has been reported. Careful monitoring during infusion is needed in order to avoid potential complications related to extravasation such as soft tissue injury, necrosis, and purple glove syndrome. A more detailed discussion about complications related to extravasation, including purple glove syndrome will be detailed later in this chapter.

With regards to distribution of phenytoin, this is perhaps the most significant pharmacological factor at play that accounts for the variability in the pediatric and neonatal population. As mentioned above, protein binding is decreased in the neonatal and pediatric population due to lower affinity for drugs, deficient albumin levels, and/or bilirubin competing for protein binding sites. This is more pronounced in the neonatal population where fetal albumin is present. Phenytoin is over 90% bound to proteins, most of which is to albumin. Decreased protein binding results in an increased phenytoin free fraction which is biologically active after distribution. The increased free fraction of phenytoin can result in toxicity and prolonged elimination. However, opposing this is the fact that the rate of renal elimination is inversely proportional to protein binding. In general, it appears the sum result of this favors toxicity over subtherapeutic dosing. Regardless, the free fraction should be considered a more accurate representation of serum levels in younger age groups. It is important to note that toxicity can occur in the face of a normal total phenytoin serum level (10-20 mg/L) which is a measurement of both bound and unbound (free) medication. The therapeutic range for free fraction of serum phenytoin is between 1-2 mg/L and increased risk for toxicity usually seen after >5 mg/mL [37].

Metabolism of phenytoin should also be considered when administering to both the neonatal and pediatric population. Phenytoin is metabolized to inactive metabolites primarily by CYP 2C9 and 2C19 [20, 40]. Specifically, CYP 2C9 and 2C19 are variability expressed during the neonatal period. 2C9 has low activity during the 1st month of life and reaches adult activity between 1 to 6 months. CYP 2C19 has minimal expression up until 2 days of birth when its expression rapidly increases, however, adult levels are not reached until 2 years of age [29, 38-43]. This variable and immature expression of certain important CYP450s can significantly alter drug metabolism and therefore increase the risk for toxicity as less parent phenytoin remains in the serum and tissue and risking cumulative dose stacking in the neonate. Additionally, as concentrations above the therapeutic range increase, phenytoin metabolism switches from 1st degree to zero-degree kinetics and therefore becomes dose dependent furthering the half-life and thus risk for toxicity. In addition to the age dependent maturation of these enzymes accounting for decreased metabolism, literature primarily restricted to the adult population evaluating the association of phenytoin toxicity in the context of CYP 2C9 and C19 polymorphisms has been cited [40, 44, 59]. In one case report that published an association between CYP 2C9 and C19 polymorphisms, claimed to be the first to make this association in the pediatric population [40]. This case reported on a 2-year-old girl with a history of cryptogenic epilepsy who developed status epilepticus and showed signs of phenytoin toxicity 2 hours after receiving her loading dose with no specific rational for toxicity including a review of drug-drug interactions and dosing. As a result, phenytoin serum levels and CYP2C9 and CYP2C19 genetic polymorphisms were sent for analysis. Her serum phenytoin level was found to be 69 mg/L (ref: 10-20 mg/L) and she was found to be homozygous for the CYP2C9*2 allele and heterozygous for the CYP2C19*4. Further research is needed to evaluate clinically relevant rates of polymorphisms and therefore potentially guide therapy in the future. At this time, CYP testing for polymorphisms is not recommended based on the lack of data. However, this illustrates the complexity of drug metabolism and the many factors which can influence drug metabolism.

## Dosing Recommendations of Phenytoin and Fosphenytoin

*Status Epilepticus - Phenytoin*: Intravenous dosing in neonates and the pediatric population does not significantly differ from adult dosing as referenced by the FDA's Parental Dilantin (Phenytoin Sodium Injection, USP) instructions. [Table 3.2]. For the pediatric dosing, the loading dose is recommended at 15-20 mg/kg IV at a rate not exceeding 1-3 mg/kg/min or 50 mg per minute, whichever is slower. In adults a lower dosage of 10-15 mg/kg IV at a rate not exceeding 50 mg per minute is recommended. The only consideration in dosing that is highlighted is the weight-based rate of infusion in order to avoid cardiovascular complications associated with phenytoin [71].

*Status Epilepticus – Fosphenytoin*: Fosphenytoin sodium injection can be administered both intravenously or intramuscularly; however, the intravenous route is the more commonly used and the recommended route as per the FDA's prescribing information [72]. As with phenytoin, administration of a loading dose is recommended parenterally in both adults and pediatrics; however, the maintenance dose is only available for the intravenous or intramuscular route and not orally. It is important to note that dosing is measured in milligram "phosphenytoin equivalents" (PE) and not in milligrams. Also, important to highlight, while fosphenytoin can cause rate related cardiovascular toxicity, the recommended rate of infusion for both the loading and maintenance dose in both populations are more liberal as compared to phenytoin [72] [Table 3.3].

*Seizures (Non-Emergent) – Phenytoin* [Tables 3.4 and 3.5]: Non-emergent treatment of seizures with phenytoin should be managed with oral therapy over the parenteral route to avoid unnecessary rate related cardiovascular complications. There are four available oral formulations: Immediate release tablets (Prompt Phenytoin Sodium capsules), extended release capsules (Dilantin Kapseal), chewable tablets (Dilantin Infatabs), and immediate release suspension (Dilantin-125). The Dilantin capsules (immediate release and extended release capsules) are the sodium salt of phenytoin; whereas, the chewable tablet form (Dilantin Infatabs) and the suspension form (Dilantin-125 suspension) are the free acid formulation. There is an approximate 8% increase in total drug content that exists in the free acid form as compared to the sodium salt formulation. Dosage adjustments and serum monitoring should be considered when switching between a sodium salt product to a free acid product (and vice versa) due to this 8% increase in drug content in the free acid form. Dosage adjustments and consideration for serum monitoring should also be made when switching between the immediate release and extended release capsules due to pharmacokinetic differences in absorption rate [73-76].

**Table 3.2. FDA's Parental dilantin (Phenytoin Sodium Injection, USP) prescribing instructions for status epilepticus in the adult and pediatric populations [71]**

| | Dosing | Recommendations | Warnings |
|---|---|---|---|
| Adults | • *Loading dose:* 10-15 mg/kg IV at a rate not exceeding 50 mg per minute<br><br>• *Maintenance Dose*: 100 mg orally or IV every 6-8 hours | • Phenytoin can be initiated with either a loading dose (followed by a maintenance infusion) or an infusion alone | • Exceeding the recommended rate of administration of increases the risk for hypotension and cardiac arrhythmias<br><br>• Cardiac monitoring is needed prior to and after administration<br><br>• Cardiovascular toxicity can still occur with Infusion rates at or below the recommended threshold rate of infusion |
| Pediatric | • *Loading dose:* 15-20 mg/kg IV at a rate not exceeding 1-3 mg/kg/min or 50 mg per minute, whichever is slower<br><br>• *Maintenance Dose:* Oral or IV every 6-8 hours | | |

**Table 3.3. FDA's Fosphenytoin sodium injection prescribing instructions for status epilepticus in the adult and pediatric populations [72]**

<table>
<tr><th></th><th>Dosing</th><th>Recommendations</th><th>Warnings</th></tr>
<tr><td>Adults</td><td>• Loading dose:<br>15-20 mg PE/kg IV at a rate of 100 to 150 mg PE/min<br><br>• Maintenance Dose:<br>4-6 mg PE/kg/day IV in divided doses at a rate no greater than 150 mg PE/min</td><td rowspan="2">• Like phenytoin, fosphenytoin should also be rate limited for both the loading and maintenance dosing intravenously, although a faster rate is acceptable.</td><td rowspan="2">• Exceeding the recommended rate of administration of increases the risk for hypotension and cardiac arrhythmias<br><br>• Cardiac monitoring is needed prior to and after administration<br><br>• Cardiovascular toxicity can still occur with Infusion rates at or below the recommended threshold rate of infusion</td></tr>
<tr><td>Pediatric</td><td>• Loading dose:<br>15 to 20 mg PE/kg IV at a rate of 2 mg PE/kg/min (or 150 mg PE/min, whichever is slower)<br><br>• Maintenance Dose:<br>2-4 mg PE/kg IV which should be given 12 hours after the loading dose and then continued every 12 hours (4 to 8 mg PE/kg/day in divided doses) at a rate of 1-2 mg PE/kg/min (or 100 mg PE/min, whichever is slower)</td></tr>
</table>

**Table 3.4. Phenytoin (oral) prescribing instructions for non-emergent seizure management in the adult population [73-76]**

| | Prompt Phenytoin Sodium Capsules (Dilantin) [73] | Extended Phenytoin Sodium Capsules (Dilantin, Kapseal) [74] | Dilantin Infatabs (chewable) [75] | Dilantin-125 Suspension [76] |
|---|---|---|---|---|
| Formulation | Sodium Salt | Sodium Salt | Free Acid | Free Acid |
| Adult Dosing | • *Initial dose:*<br>100 mg three times daily, individualize dosage with dosage adjustments at no less than 7- to 10-day intervals.<br><br>• *Maintenance dose:*<br>300 to 400 mg/day; an increase to 600 mg/day may be necessary. | • *Initial dose:*<br>One gram divided in three doses: 400 mg, 300 mg, 300 mg, administered in two-hour intervals. Maintenance dosing initiated 24 hrs after loading dose.<br><br>• *Maintenance Dose:*<br>– Divided daily dosage:<br>– Starting dose - One 100-mg capsule three times daily (dosage then adjusted to suite individual requirements)<br>– Once-a-day dosage:<br>– One 300-mg capsule once daily | • *Starting dosage:*<br>Two 50-mg Infatabs three times daily | • *Starting dosage:*<br>One teaspoonful (5 mL) three times daily (dosage then adjusted to suite individual requirements) |
| Comments (Adults) | | • *Initial Dose:*<br>– Should be considered only in patients that require more rapid steady-state serum levels where the intravenous route is less desirable | | |

**Table 3.4. (Continued)**

| | Prompt Phenytoin Sodium Capsules (Dilantin) [73] | Extended Phenytoin Sodium Capsules (Dilantin, Kapseal) [74] | Dilantin Infatabs (chewable) [75] | Dilantin-125 Suspension [76] |
|---|---|---|---|---|
| Comments (Adults) | | – Should be restricted to clinics or hospitals where serum concentration monitoring is feasible<br>– Should NOT be used for patients with a history of hepatic and/or renal disease<br><br>• Maintenance - divided daily dosage:<br>– The divided daily dosage is indicated for patients who received no prior treatment<br>– Most adults require one 100-mg capsule three to four times daily<br><br>• Maintenance - once-a-day dosage:<br>– Indicated for adults whose seizures are controlled on divided doses of three 100-mg capsules daily<br>– Once-a-day dosage should be especially considered for certain populations: Non-compliant patients and healthcare providers administering phenytoin to institutionalized patients. | • The recommended starting dosage is for adults who received no prior treatment<br>• Dose adjustments can be made up to a maximum of twelve Infatabs (600 mg) per day | • The recommended starting dosage is for adults who received no prior treatment<br>• If necessary, dosage can be increased to five teaspoonfuls daily |

**Table 3.5. Phenytoin (oral) prescribing instructions for non-emergent seizure management in the pediatric population [73-76]**

| | Prompt Phenytoin Sodium Capsules (Dilantin) [73] | Extended Phenytoin Sodium Capsules (Dilantin, Kapseal) [74] | Dilantin Infatabs (chewable) [75] | Dilantin-125 Suspension [76] |
|---|---|---|---|---|
| Formulation | Sodium Salt | Sodium Salt | Free Acid | Free Acid |
| Pediatric Dosing | • Initial Dose: 5 mg/kg/day in two or three equally divided doses<br>• Maintenance Dose: Typically, in the range of 4-8 mg/kg/day orally; not to exceed 300 mg/day. Dose adjustments to be made prior to 7-10 days. | | | |
| Comments (Pediatrics) | • Children > 6 years old may require the minimum adult dose (300 mg/day)<br>• Daily maintenance dosage recommendation is usually 4 to 8 mg/kg | | | |

**Table 3.6. FDA's fosphenytoin sodium injection instructions for non-emergent seizure management in the adult and pediatric populations [72]**

<table>
<tr><th></th><th>Dosing</th><th>Recommendations</th><th>Warnings</th></tr>
<tr><td>Adults</td><td>• Loading dose:<br>10-20 mg PE/kg given IV or IM<br><br>• Maintenance Dose:<br>4 to 6 mg PE/kg/day IV in divided doses at a rate no greater than 150 mg PE/min</td><td rowspan="2">• Like phenytoin, fosphenytoin administration should also be rate limited for both the loading and maintenance dosing intravenously, although a faster rate is acceptable.</td><td rowspan="2">• Exceeding the recommended rate of administration of increases the risk for hypotension and cardiac arrhythmias<br><br>• Cardiac monitoring is needed prior to and after administration<br><br>• Cardiovascular toxicity can still occur with Infusion rates at or below the recommended threshold rate of infusion</td></tr>
<tr><td>Pediatric</td><td>• Loading dose:<br>10-15 mg PE/kg IV at a rate of 2 mg PE/kg/min<br>(or 150 mg PE/min, whichever is slower)<br><br>• Maintenance Dose:<br>2 to 4 mg PE/kg which should be given 12 hours after the loading dose and then continued every 12 hours (4 to 8 mg PE/kg/day in divided doses) at a rate of 1 to 2 mg PE/kg/min (or 100 mg PE/min, whichever is slower)</td></tr>
</table>

*Seizures (Non-Emergent) – Fosphenytoin*

For non-emergent seizure management, fosphenytoin can be started as a loading dose in both populations. The loading dose in adults can be given either IV or IM. However, the IM dose is generally not recommended and dosing is not provided by the FDA dosing instructions for pediatric populations. In general, the FDA recommends using oral phenytoin over fosphenytoin for which no oral dosing is available, for the management of non-emergent seizures in order to avoid potential cardiovascular complications related to the intravenous administration of fosphenytoin [72].

## Adverse Effects in the Neonatal and Pediatric Population

Phenytoin use has a narrow therapeutic window lending to the risk for toxicity which presents predominately with CNS manifestations such as altered mental status, nystagmus, ataxia, to name a few. In addition to toxicity relating to overdose either intentional, exploratory, iatrogenic, or inadvertent, some adverse effects are not related and/or chronic manifestations. See chapter 2 for detailed descriptions of these adverse effects and toxicities; in this next section a few selected adverse effects which deserve special attention as they relate to the neonatal and pediatric population will be highlighted.

## Extravasation and Purple Glove Syndrome

As mentioned earlier in this chapter, special attention is needed to the intravenous administration of phenytoin as it relates to the risk for extravasation with the potential for serious soft tissue destruction. With smaller diameter veins, extravasation is more likely in the pediatric and neonatal population as compared to adults. It is important to not only ensure adequate cannulation prior to administration but also to evaluate for signs of extravasation and local toxicity throughout the infusion. While phenytoin is a weak acid, its vehicle is alkaline. Phenytoin carrier is sodium hydroxide while its vehicle is composed of both ethanol and propylene glycol [1]. As a result, extravasation can result in serious soft tissue and vascular damage from necrosis secondary to these irritating substances. On the other hand, fosphenytoin is less likely to cause significant local toxicity as it is water soluble in its vehicle, with a pH of 8.6-9 [1]. While fosphenytoin is generally regarded as less irritating, there have been some reports of significant toxicity related to purple glove syndrome (PGS) [45-47]. In one prospective study by Appleton and Gill in 2003, the type and rate of IV phenytoin adverse effects were evaluated [1]. The study involved 22 children who received a total of 100 doses over a 10-month period. They found that 27% (n = 6) suffered at least one adverse effect which among cardiovascular toxicity included extravasation from either infiltrated or clogged cannulas. Extravasation accounted for 3 patients and occlusion of the IV accounted for 2 patients. Interestingly, none of these patients demonstrated signs of significant local toxicity including skin discoloration, ulceration, or signs of PGS. In a review by Garbovsky et al, PGS was evaluated in all age populations [48]. They found 82 cases of parenteral phenytoin induced PGS and 5 cases of fosphenytoin induced PGS from 1984 to 2015. Here they found 8 (9.8%) of the total cases to be pediatric patients. While toxicity is a concern for phenytoin and likely to a lesser degree fosphenytoin, the rates of significant local injury including PGS is likely rare but clinicians should be aware of these potentially devastating complications when administering parenteral phenytoin/fosphenytoin.

## DRESS Syndrome

Drug-induced hypersensitivity or Drug Reaction with Eosinophilia and Systemic Symptom (DRESS) is a relatively uncommon complication from a variety of medications, most importantly cyclic anticonvulsants. This syndrome could be difficult to identify. While the prevalence of DRESS syndrome is more in adults as compared to the pediatric population, special attention is warranted due to the difficulty in diagnosis and significant morbidity and mortality associated with this syndrome [49]. DRESS syndrome is an idiosyncratic reaction characterized multi-organ involvement, fever, and cutaneous findings. It is most associated with aromatic anticonvulsants such as phenytoin, phenobarbital, and carbamazepine [49, 50]. The incidence in children is not well established and no clinical control studies regarding treatment for DRESS specific to the pediatric population exists [50]. In the general population, the incidence of DRESS secondary to anticonvulsants is in the rage of 1/1000 to 1/10,000. Again, the incidence in children is not known but likely less prevalent compared to adults [50-52]. The average age in children who develop this syndrome is around 9 years old which is based on retrospective studies [52, 53]. In a study by Newell et al. 32 pediatric patients diagnosed with anticonvulsant hypersensitivity syndrome were retrospectively studied [50]. Here they found that the mean duration of therapy prior to onset of symptoms was 3 weeks. Phenytoin, carbamazepine, and phenobarbital were the most common implicated medications in the study. With regards to presentation, fever and rash were present in all patients, lymphadenopathy in 84.4%, hematological finings in 93.8%, and hepatic involvement in 90.4%. These findings are closely related to adult presentation with fever and rash being almost universally present.

## Gingival Hyperplasia

Hyperplasia of the gums is a relatively common chronic adverse effect of phenytoin which can present as mild mucosal outgrowth of the gingiva to significant hyperplasia requiring dental correction [54]. Although a variety of medications can cause this condition, phenytoin has been the most classically described medication responsible [54]. Further, it is estimated that up to half of patients on chronic phenytoin therapy develop gingival hypertrophy in the general population and it is more common in children as compared to adults [54-56]. The onset of symptoms often occurs within the first 3 months, and once developed tends to reach a state of equilibrium by one year from symptom onset [54, 57]. While this is not a life threatening condition, given its prevalence amongst patients on phenytoin and its increased incidence in children and adolescence, clinicians should be aware of this very common adverse effect and refer patients to dentistry for further management. In some case of extreme refractory hyperplasia, patients may require gingivectomy when meticulous cleaning has been exhausted.

## Phenytoin Toxicity: Pediatric and Neonatal Presentation, History and Physical Examination Considerations

In general phenytoin toxicity presents similarly in all age groups in terms of organ system involvement. In all age groups, central nervous system toxicity is the most common presentation of severe toxicity. Cerebellar and vestibular toxicity are the hallmarks of phenytoin toxicity. In adults, serum phenytoin levels closely correlate with signs of toxicity. [Table 3.7].

**Table 3.7. Signs and symptoms correlating to serum phenytoin concentrations**

| Serum Phenytoin Concentration | Signs/Symptoms |
|---|---|
| 10 to 20 mg/L | Therapeutic, rare effects |
| 20 to 30 mg/L | Nystagmus |
| 30 to 40 mg/L | Ataxia, tremor, slurred speech |
| 40 to 50 mg/L | Altered mental status, confusion, lethargy |
| >50 mg/L | Coma, seizures, death |

As discussed above, in the neonatal and younger infant population, using total serum phenytoin levels may not accurately reflect true serum levels. Toxicity in this population can occur despite total serum level within the therapeutic range. Therefore, a more accurate serum level is by obtaining the free (unbound level) which reflects more accurately true serum concentration thereby reducing toxicity with the appropriate dosing corrections. In considering the physical examination in neonates and infants, classical signs such as ataxia and slurred speech will not be as apparent as in adults, depending on the developmental stage of the. Therefore, awareness of the full clinical spectrum of phenytoin toxicity is necessary to avoid misdiagnosis.

## Treatment Considerations of Phenytoin Toxicity in the Neonatal and Pediatric Population

In general, specific to the neonatal and pediatric populations, the treatment of phenytoin toxicity is relatively similar to the methods used in the adult population. There is no antidote available, and for much of the literature of gastrointestinal decontamination, limited evidence supports improved outcome [58]. While so, activated charcoal should be considered in cases where significant toxicity is expected which may be the case in an intentional overdose with a known mg/kg ingestion or patients presenting with signs of toxicity. While earlier administration of activated charcoal is ideal, consideration for more distant ingestions should be made in cases of prolonged toxicity. Multi-dose activated charcoal (MDAC) should also be considered but evidence is lacking to strongly support its use and evidence is primarily based on case reports and experimental studies [58, 59]. In a case report by Chan et al. three patients who were phenytoin toxic with known CYP 2C9 polymorphisms, 2 of the 3 patients were treated with MDAC resulting in rapid reductions of phenytoin serum levels as compared to the single patient who did not receive MDAC [59]. Interestingly, all three patients had not received phenytoin for over 40 hours prior to MDAC administration. Provided none of these patients had suspected intentional overdoses and thus no concern for significant gut burden, the use of MDAC potentially was helpful secondary to "gut dialysis." The potential benefit of MDAC relating to gastrointestinal recirculation was suggested by a volunteer study conducted by Mauro et al. in 1987. Seven healthy volunteers received 15 mg/kg intravenous phenytoin with and without activated charcoal. A total of 300 grams were administered in repeated doses over a

2-day time window. They determined that serum half-life decreased from 44.5 to 22.3 hours in the charcoal group [61]. In another case report, a 36-year-old male who presented with phenytoin toxicity secondary to hepatitis was administered MDAC for a total of 4 doses which brought his serum level from 43 mg/L to therapeutic range within 36 hours [60].

Whole bowel irrigation may be a viable option especially in cases of extended release products or cases where co-ingestions known to decrease GI motility are present, such as anticholinergics.

Finally, enhanced methods of elimination such as plasmapheresis, hemodialysis, or hemoperfusion, have not been shown to be effective in outcome with the limited data on the neonatal and pediatric populations [2, 58]. Most evidence on these enhanced elimination techniques is primarily anecdotal. However, recommendations set forth by EXTRIP (extracorporeal treatments in poisoning) workgroup which is data obtained by expert panels with recommendations based on systemic reviews.[62] Recommendations are as follows: (1) Intermittent hemodialysis (HD) is the preferred ECTR in phenytoin poisoning (Level 1, Class D recommendation); (2) Intermittent hemoperfusion (HP) is an acceptable alternative if intermittent HD is not available (Level 1, Class D recommendation); (3) Indications for ECTR: Prolonged coma is expected or present, prolonged incapacitating ataxia is present or expected, recommend against ECTR based on suspected dose of phenytoin alone or phenytoin serum levels alone. It is important to note that these studies are not specific to the population of interest in this chapter but provides the most systematically evaluated recommendations based on available literature. Therefore, the above should also be considered in the pediatric and neonatal populations considering the risks versus benefits of more invasive therapies.

## SPECIAL CONSIDERATIONS IN POPULATIONS WITH HEPATIC OR RENAL IMPAIRMENTS

Hepatic and/or renal impairment can have serious clinical implications for patients who take medications that are dependent on both of these organs for metabolism and/or elimination. For example, the liver is primarily responsible for the metabolism of many drugs in order to produce inactive metabolites ready for elimination in conjunction with other processes. Some medications are metabolized into more active or potent compounds relative to the parent compound (e.g., codeine metabolism to morphine), others converted into the active form (e.g., fosphenytoin to phenytoin; clopidogrel to 2-oxo-clopidogrel) named prodrugs, while others are converted in a number of inactive metabolites. In addition to modification of the parent compound, the hepatobiliary system within itself eliminates drug from the body. While the kidneys may directly or indirectly influence the metabolism of drugs, elimination of parent and/or active/inactive metabolites serves as the kidney's primary role. Commonly, the liver and kidney work in sync within one another to metabolize and eliminate drug. This system is not static but rather dynamic and begins immediately after absorption [63]. In addition to effects on metabolism and elimination, dysfunction in both organs can lead to disruption in the distribution of drugs. For example, carrier proteins such as albumin are created in the liver and a deficiency in these proteins can lead to decreased protein binding and therefore greater fraction of active (unbound) drug. This can lead to toxicity even with 'therapeutic' dosages in the general population [63, 64]. Renal insufficiency can lead to altered protein binding from hypoalbuminemia, drug-drug interactions, and uremia [65].

Phenytoin is a medication that can be significantly affected by dysfunction in either of these two organs. Perhaps the most important consideration is patients with hypoalbuminemia. Again, this can result from either hepatic and/or renal disease, however, hypoalbuminemia is a relatively common condition with a reported incidence of up to 50% of the population [66]. Phenytoin has a large volume of distribution (0.7 L/kg) and roughly 90% protein bound with albumin and 10% the free or active form. The plasma half-life ranges from 6 to 24 hours at therapeutic plasma concentration (10–20 mg/L). However, with hepatic/renal impairment, saturation elimination kinetics may occur within the total phenytoin therapeutic range. Saturation of enzymes responsible for metabolism will result in a shift from first order to zero order kinetics [55]. This shift from concentration dependent elimination (first order) to fixed mg per unit time elimination (zero order) will result in a prolonged elimination half-life. Therefore, a more accurate measure of clinically relevant active phenytoin is the free fraction (unbound), the pharmacologically active fraction. As such is the case with the neonatal population, clinical toxicity can occur within the 'therapeutic' range of total serum phenytoin levels. Therefore, clinicians should consider this laboratory assessment as the more accurate means in determining levels in order to tailor necessary dosage adjustment and to avoid potential toxicity. These considerations hold true for both patient populations with hepatic or renal disease secondary to hypoalbuminemia.

Patients with liver disease may also have some degree of altered metabolism. As discussed in the neonatal/pediatric population section, phenytoin is metabolized extensively by the CYP 450 system to inactive metabolites [20, 40]. The primary inactive metabolite via hepatic CYP 2C9 and C19 oxidation is hydroxyphenytoin (5-(4'-hydroxyphenyl)-5-phenylhydantoin or p-HPPH) [67, 68]. This para-hydroxylated inactive metabolite is further metabolized via hepatic glucuronidation before excretion in the urine. Important to note, preceding p-HPPH formation is the formation of an active arene oxide intermediate which has traditionally been associated with a variety of idiosyncratic reactions which will be touched on below [67, 69]. Patients with liver impairment are at risk for developing phenytoin toxicity due to the inability to hydroxylate phenytoin to its hydroxyphenytoin inactive metabolite (p-HPPH). This results in increased serum phenytoin concentration and the risk for the development of toxicity. Therefore, patients with liver disease are more susceptible to supratherapeutic phenytoin concentrations resulting in toxicity secondary alterations in protein binding and/or inability to metabolize phenytoin.

While patients may experience toxicity directly due to liver or kidney disease can occur, it is important to evaluate all potential causes of toxicity. For example, patients who have milder forms of liver disease may still have intact functioning of the CYP enzyme system. Other causes in this context may include unintentional or intentional overdose, polymorphisms in metabolism, co-ingestants of certain foods and medications [see Chapter 5] and idiosyncratic reactions unrelated to dose. Dose-related toxicity occurs secondary to failure a failure in distribution (faulty or decreased protein binding), metabolism (p-hydroxylation of phenytoin via CYP 2C9 and 2C19), and/or excretion (hepatic or renal disease).

While idiosyncratic reactions are adverse effects, they are not dose-dependent and unrelated to increased phenytoin concentration [67]. The most notable idiosyncratic reactions associated with phenytoin are anticonvulsant hypersensitivity syndrome, DRESS, Stevens- Johnson Syndrome (SJS)/Toxic-Epidermal Necrolysis (TEN), and hepatoxicity [67]. As mentioned above, the hydroxylation of phenytoin to its major inactive metabolite, pHHH is preceded by a reactive intermediate. This reactive compound is an arene-oxide intermediate. In normal circumstances, this intermediate is further metabolized to phenytoin dihydrodiol via the enzyme epoxide hydrolase. It is thought that deficiency in this enzyme is responsible, at least in part, for the development of these idiosyncratic reactions. Formation of the arene-oxide group requires an aromatic ring explaining why only some anticonvulsants are associated with this adverse reaction.

In addition to the consideration of non-dose related causes for phenytoin toxicity, polymorphisms in both CYP2C9 and 2C19 resulting in slow metabolism should also be considered. This is especially true in the context of prolonged toxicity with no logical explanation. As mentioned in the pediatric/neonatal section, literature on polymorphism disrupting hepatic metabolism has been documented mainly in the adult population [40, 44, 59]. While obtaining specialized testing such as genetic studies is by no means necessary in most cases, considerations should be made in the context of uncertain situations especially in the context of exaggerated and prolonged toxicity/phenytoin levels.

With regards to specific recommendations on dosing algorithms in these two populations, there is no specific gold standard method or any evidenced based approaches. However, some caution is warranted. It is perhaps most important to be cognizant that patients with hepatic and/or renal disease have a higher propensity for the development of toxicity on top of an already narrow therapeutic index. Therefore, it is important to tailor therapy on an individual basis. Perhaps more frequent monitoring of serum concentration levels in these populations is best. Due to saturable kinetics resulting in toxicity even with therapeutic range total phenytoin levels, a free phenytoin (unbound) level is most ideal in this population for more accurate assessment of true serum concentrations. Also, patients with hepatic and/or renal disease should be closely monitored in cases where loading dosages are advised. However, caution should be advised when deciding to use off-label dosing in both of these populations, as the FDA recommends against an oral loading dose when treating non-emergent seizure disorders.

## Conclusion

It is critical for healthcare providers to be aware of the limitations and precautions of phenytoin's use when managing special populations. Relevant to this chapter, the neonatal/pediatric age group and populations that are inflicted with hepatic or kidney disease are susceptible to the development of phenytoin toxicity and therefore a strategic approach to the management of these populations should be instituted.

This chapter highlighted the relevant pharmacokinetic profiles specific to the neonatal and pediatric populations. With knowledge of these differences, providers can incorporate a more tailored approach as a whole to the neonatal and pediatric populations. As we have discussed, dramatic pharmacokinetic and pharmacodynamic differences exists even between the neonate and infant. While weight-based dosing is based on best evidence for the pediatric population at large, considerations for possible dosing adjustments and serum concentration monitoring should be considered between the premature neonate, term neonate, young infant all the way to adolescence. This poses a significant challenge in the careful administration of phenytoin to these younger age groups. However, with a patient-specific approach to phenytoin dosing, serum concentration monitoring, and knowledge of the signs and symptoms consistent with phenytoin toxicity, providers can increase the likelihood for therapeutic success while decreasing the chance for toxicity. Lastly, this chapter reviewed age-specific adverse effects that have a propensity to afflict specific age groups. Therefore, an understanding of these specific adverse effects can increase the likelihood for avoiding these effects or halting the progression of an adverse effect in its earlier stages. This chapter hopefully provided an awareness of the susceptibility of the neonatal and pediatric populations and provided practical information for an age-specific tailored approach for the administration of phenytoin/fosphenytoin.

With regards to those with liver or kidney disease, management can be especially difficult considering the lack of specific evidence-based dosing algorithms which leaves the provider more dependent on clinical judgement and personal experience. Therefore, while dosage adjustments should still be considered, the reliance on both strict serum concentration monitoring and clinical evaluation for signs/symptoms of toxicity is critical in reducing the likelihood for toxicity. Additionally, decisions such as avoiding unnecessary intravenous and oral loading, particularly for the management of non-emergent seizures, could potentially decrease the chances for toxicity. In cases of status epilepticus, clinical judgement should be used when deciding if loading doses are necessary and if so consideration for dosage adjustments should be made. The approach to this should be considered on a case-by-case basis weighing the risk of continued seizures to the risk of potential toxicity with full loading doses.

For all patients, avoiding intravenous dosing when oral dosing is sufficient will eliminate the risk of rate related cardiovascular complications caused by the intravenous route for both phenytoin and fosphenytoin. When intravenous administration is indicated, adhering strictly to the appropriate recommended rates of infusion set forth by the FDA will significantly decrease rate-related cardiovascular toxicity. Perhaps equally important for the avoidance of phenytoin toxicity is using one's clinical judgement with regards to considering an alternative anti-convulsant that may be better suited for an individual. With newer generation anti-convulsant therapies currently being prescribed today and many with more favorable toxicological profiles as compared to phenytoin, weighing the risks and benefits for their use as an alternative should be in the forefront of one's clinical decision making in order to optimize best outcomes.

## References

[1] Appleton RE1, Gill A. Adverse events associated with intravenous phenytoin in children: a prospective study. *Seizure.* 2003 Sep; 12(6):369-72. PMID: 12915082.

[2] Iorga A, Horowitz BZ. Phenytoin Toxicity. [Updated 2019 Feb 28]. In: *StatPearls* [Internet]. Treasure Island (FL): StatPearls Publishing; 2019 Jan-. Available from: https://www.ncbi.nlm.nih.gov/books/NBK482444/.

[3] Bashiri FA. Childhood epilepsies: What should a pediatrician know? Neurosciences (Riyadh). 2017 Jan; 22(1):14-19. doi: 10.17712/nsj.2017.1.20160244. PubMed PMID: 28064325; *PubMed Central* PMCID: PMC5726831.

[4] Camfield P, Camfield C. Incidence, prevalence and aetiology of seizures and epilepsy in children. *Epileptic Disord.* 2015; 17:117–123.

[5] Slaughter LA, Patel AD, Slaughter JL. Pharmacological treatment of neonatal seizures: a systematic review. J Child Neurol. 2013 Mar;28(3):351-64. doi: 10.1177/0883073812470734. Epub 2013 Jan 14. PubMed PMID: 23318696; *PubMed Central PMCID*: PMC3805825.

[6] Lanska MJ, Lanska DJ, Baumann RJ, Kryscio RJ. A population-based study of neonatal seizures in Fayette County, Kentucky. *Neurology.* 1995;45:724–732. [PubMed] [Google Scholar].

[7] Ronen GM, Penney S, Andrews W. The epidemiology of clinical neonatal seizures in Newfoundland: a population-based study. *J Pediatr.* 1999;134:71–75. [PubMed] [Google Scholar].

[8] Saliba RM, Annegers JF, Waller DK, et al. Incidence of neonatal seizures in Harris County, Texas, 1992–1994. *Am J Epidemiol.* 1999;150:763–769.

[9] Tekgul H, Gauvreau K, Soul J, Murphy L, Robertson R, Stewart J, et al. The current etiologic profile and neurodevelopmental outcome of seizures in term newborn infants. *Pediatrics.* 2006;117:1270–80.

[10] Painter MJ, Scher MS, Stein AD, et al. Phenobarbital compared with phenytoin for the treatment of neonatal seizures. *N Engl J Med.* 1999;341:485–489.

[11] Ku LC, Smith PB. Dosing in neonates: special considerations in physiology and trial design. Pediatr Res. 2015 Jan;77(1-1):2-9. doi: 10.1038/pr.2014.143. Epub 2014 Sep 30. PubMed PMID: 25268145; *PubMed Central* PMCID: PMC4268272.

[12] Kimland E, Odlind V. Off-label drug use in pediatric patients. *Clin Pharmacol Ther. 2012*;91:796–801.

[13] Boylan G, Rennie J, Chorley G, et al. Second-line anticonvulsant treatment of neonatal seizures. *Neurology.* 2004;62:486–488.

[14] Silverstein FS, Ferriero DM. Off-label use of antiepileptic drugs for the treatment of neonatal seizures. *Pediatr Neurol.* 2008;39:77–79.

[15] Ahmad KA1,2, Desai SJ3, Bennett MM4, Ahmad SF2, Ng YT2, Clark RH5, Tolia VN6,7. Changing antiepileptic drug use for seizures in US neonatal intensive care units from 2005 to 2014. *J Perinatol.* 2017 Mar;37(3):296-300. doi: 10.1038/jp.2016.206. Epub 2016 Nov 10. PMID: 27831551 doi: 10.1038/jp.2016.206.

[16] Trends in Antiepileptic Drug Use in Children and Adolescents With Epilepsy. Liu X., Carney P. R., Bussing R., Segal R., Cottler L. B., Winterstein A. G. (2017) *Pediatric Neurology,* 74, pp. 32-40. PMID: 28676250 doi: 10.1016/j.pediatrneurol.2017.05.016.

[17] Moavero R1,2, Pisani LR3, Pisani F4, Curatolo P1. Safety and tolerability profile of new antiepileptic drug treatment in children with epilepsy. *Expert Opin Drug Saf.* 2018 Oct;17(10):1015-1028. doi: 10.1080/14740338.2018.1518427. Epub 2018 Sep 17. PMID: 30169997.

[18] Fernandez E, Perez R, Hernandez A, Tejada P, Arteta M, Ramos JT. Factors and Mechanisms for Pharmacokinetic Differences between Pediatric Population and Adults. *Pharmaceutics.* 2011 Feb 7;3(1):53-

72. doi: 10.3390/pharmaceutics3010053. PubMed PMID: 24310425; PubMed Central PMCID: PMC3857037.

[19] Eva Fernandez, Raul Perez, Alfredo Hernandez, Pilar Tejada, Marta Arteta, Jose T. Ramos. *Pharmaceutics.* 2011 Mar; 3(1): 53–72. Published online 2011 Feb 7. doi: 10.3390/pharmaceutics3010053 PMCID: PMC3857037.

[20] Clinical pharmacokinetics in newborns and infants. Age-related differences and therapeutic implications. Morselli PL, Franco-Morselli R, Bossi L. *Clin Pharmacokinet.* 1980 Nov-Dec; 5(6):485-527.

[21] Guidelines on paediatric dosing on the basis of developmental physiology and pharmacokinetic considerations. Bartelink IH, Rademaker CM, Schobben AF, van den Anker JN. *Clin Pharmacokinet.* 2006; 45(11):1077-97.

[22] Strolin Benedetti M, Baltes EL. Drug metabolism and disposition in children. *Fundam Clin Pharmacol.* 2003 Jun; 17(3):281-99.

[23] Pharmacologic evaluation of orally administered antibiotics in infants and children: effect of feeding on bioavailability. McCracken GH Jr, Ginsburg CM, Clahsen JC, Thomas ML. *Pediatrics.* 1978 Nov; 62(5):738-43.

[24] Strolin Benedetti M, Whomsley R, Baltes EL. Differences in absorption, distribution, metabolism and excretion of xenobiotics between the paediatric and adult populations. *Expert Opin Drug Metab Toxicol.* 2005 Oct; 1(3):447-71.

[25] Bile acid concentrations in serum and duodenal aspirates of healthy preterm infants: effects of gestational and postnatal age. Boehm G, Braun W, Moro G, Minoli I. *Biol Neonate.* 1997; 71(4):207-14.

[26] Saavedra I., Quinones L., Saavedra M., Sasso J., Leon J., Roco A. Farmacocinetica de medicamentos de uso pediatrico, vision actual. *Rev. Chil. Pediatr.* 2008;79:249–258.

[27] Koren G. Therapeutic drug monitoring principles in the neonate. *National Academy of Clinical Biochemistry Clin Chem.* 1997 Jan; 43(1):222-7.

[28] American Academy of Pediatrics. Committee on Drugs. Alternative routes of drug administration–advantages and disadvantages (subject review) *Pediatrics.* 1997;100:143–152.

[29] Ku LC, Smith PB. Dosing in neonates: special considerations in physiology and trial design. *Pediatr Res.* 2015 Jan;77(1-1):2-9. doi: 10.1038/pr.2014.143. Epub 2014 Sep 30. PubMed PMID: 25268145; *PubMed Central* PMCID: PMC4268272.

[30] Kearns GL, Abdel-Rahman SM, Alander SW, Blowey DL, Leeder JS, Kauffman RE. Developmental pharmacology--drug disposition, action, and therapy in infants and children. *N Engl J Med.* 2003 Sep 18; 349(12):1157-67.

[31] Allegaert K, Verbesselt R, Naulaers G, et al. Developmental pharmacology: neonates are not just small adults. *Acta Clin Belg.* 2008; 63:16–24.

[32] Warner A. Drug use in the neonate: interrelationships of pharmacokinetics, toxicity, and biochemical maturity. *Clin Chem.* 1986; 32:721–7.

[33] Seyberth HW, Kauffman RE. Basics and dynamics of neonatal and pediatric pharmacology. *Handb Exp Pharmacol.* 2011; 205():3-49.

[34] Tayman C, Rayyan M, Allegaert K. Neonatal pharmacology: extensive interindividual variability despite limited size. *J Pediatr Pharmacol Ther.* 2011 Jul; 16(3):170-84.

[35] Smits A, Annaert P, Allegaert K. Drug disposition and clinical practice in neonates: cross talk between developmental physiology and pharmacology. *Int J Pharm.* 2013 Aug 16; 452(1-2):8-13.

[36] Vieux R, Hascoet JM, Merdariu D, Fresson J, Guillemin F. Glomerular filtration rate reference values in very preterm infants. *Pediatrics.* 2010 May; 125(5):e1186-92.

[37] Anseeuw K, Mowry JB, Burdmann EA, Ghannoum M, Hoffman RS, Gosselin S, et al. Extracorporeal treatment in phenytoin poisoning: Systematic review and recommendations from the EXTRIP (extracorporeal treatments in poisoning) workgroup. *Am J Kidney Dis.* 2015:pii: S0272-638601258-5.

[38] Seyberth HW, Kauffman RE. Basics and dynamics of neonatal and pediatric pharmacology. *Handb Exp Pharmacol*. 2011; 205():3-49.

[39] Blake MJ, Castro L, Leeder JS, Kearns GL. Ontogeny of drug metabolizing enzymes in the neonate. *Semin Fetal Neonatal Med.* 2005 Apr; 10(2):123-38.

[40] Kearns GL, Abdel-Rahman SM, Alander SW, Blowey DL, Leeder JS, Kauffman RE. Developmental pharmacology—drug disposition, action, and therapy in infants and children. *N Engl J Med.* 2003;349:1157–67.

[41] Skinner AV. Neonatal pharmacology. *Anaesth Intensive Care Med.* 2011;12:79–84.

[42] Kearns GL. Impact of developmental pharmacology on pediatric study design: overcoming the challenges. *J Allergy Clin Immunol.* 2000; 106:S128–38.

[43] Blake MJ, Castro L, Leeder JS, Kearns GL. Ontogeny of drug metabolizing enzymes in the neonate. *Semin Fetal Neonatal Med.* 2005; 10:123–38.

[44] Dorado P1, López-Torres E, Peñas-Lledó EM, Martínez-Antón J, Llerena A. Neurological toxicity after phenytoin infusion in a pediatric patient with epilepsy: influence of CYP2C9, CYP2C19 and ABCB1 genetic polymorphisms. *Pharmacogenomics J.* 2013 Aug;13(4):359-61. doi: 10.1038/tpj.2012.19. Epub 2012 May 29. PMID: 22641027 doi: 10.1038/tpj.2012.19.

[45] Purple Glove Syndrome after Phenytoin or Fosphenytoin Administration: Review of Reported Cases and Recommendations for Prevention. Lyudmila A. Garbovsky, Byron C. Drumheller, Jeanmarie Perrone. *J Med Toxicol.* 2015 Dec; 11(4): 445–459. Published online 2015 Jul 2. doi: 10.1007/s13181-015-0490-z. PMCID: PMC4675605.

[46] Cerebyx (Fosphenytoin Sodium Injection) [prescribing information]. Pfizer Labs: New York. Revised April 2014. http://labeling.pfizer.com/ShowLabeling.aspx?id=749. Accessed 6 June 2015.

[47] *Intravenous Phenytoin and Fosphenytoin Safety Concerns Background Package*. Available at: http://www.fda.gov/ downloads/

advisorycommittees/committeesmeetingmaterials/drugs/peripheralandcentralnervoussystemdrugsadvisorycommittee/ucm231776.pdf.

[48] Garbovsky LA, Drumheller BC, Perrone J. Purple Glove Syndrome after Phenytoin or Fosphenytoin Administration: Review of Reported Cases and Recommendations for Prevention. *J Med Toxicol.* 2015 Dec;11(4):445-59. doi: 10.1007/s13181-015-0490-z. PubMed PMID: 26135797; *PubMed Central* PMCID: PMC4675605.

[49] Nissrine EL Omairi, Sanae Abourazzak, Sanae Chaouki, Samir Atmani, Moustapha Hida. Drug Reaction with Eosinophilia and Systemic Symptom (DRESS) induced by carbamazepine: a case report and literature review. *Pan Afr Med J.* 2014; 18: 9. Published online 2014 May 2. doi: 10.11604/pamj.2014.18.9.3799. PMCID: PMC4213523.

[50] Mori, Francesca, Carlo Caffarelli, Silvia Caimmi, Paolo Bottau, Lucia Liotti, Fabrizio Franceschini, Fabio Cardinale, Roberto Bernardini, Giuseppe Crisafulli, Francesca Saretta, and Elio Novembre. 2019. "Drug Reaction With Eosinophilia and Systemic Symptoms (DRESS) in Children." *Acta Bio Medica Atenei Parmensis* 90 (3-S), 66-79.

[51] Chang DKM, Shear NH (1992) Cutaneous reaction to antiepileptics. *Semin Neurol* 12:329-337.

[52] Kardaun SH, Sekula P, Valeyrie-Allanore L, et al. Drug re-action with eosinophilia and systemic symptoms (DRESS): an original multisystem adverse drug reaction. Results from the prospective RegiSCAR study. *Br J Dermatol* 2013; 169: 1071-80.

[53] Newell B, Moinfar M, Mancini A, Nopper A. Retrospective analysis of 32 pediatric patients with anticonvulsant hyper-sensitivity syndrome (ACHSS). *Pediatr Dermatol* 2009; 26: 536-46.

[54] Corrêa JD, Queiroz-Junior CM, Costa JE, Teixeira AL, Silva TA. Phenytoin-induced gingival overgrowth: a review of the molecular, immune, and inflammatory features. *ISRN Dent.* 2011;2011:497850. doi: 10.5402/2011/497850. Epub 2011 Jul 25. PubMed PMID: 21991476; PubMed Central PMCID: PMC3168966.

[55] Kumar R, Singh RK, Verma N, et al. Phenytoin-induced severe gingival overgrowth in a child Case Reports 2014; 2014:bcr2014204046.

[56] Modéer T, Domeij H, Andurén I, Mustafa M, Brunius G. Effect of phenytoin on the production of interleukin-6 and interleukin-8 in human gingival fibroblasts. *Journal of Oral Pathology and Medicine*. 2000;29(10):491–499.

[57] Lin K, Guilhoto LM, Yacubian EMT. Drug-induced gingival enlargement—part II. Antiepileptic drugs: not only phenytoin is involved. *Journal of Epilepsy and Clinical Neurophysiology*. 2007;13(2):83–88.

[58] Shukla A, Sankar J, Verma A, Dubey N. Acute phenytoin intoxication in a 4-year-old mimicking viral meningoencephalitis. *BMJ Case Rep.* 2013 Jun 25;2013:bcr2013009492. doi: 10.1136/bcr-2013-009492. PubMed PMID: 23814089; *PubMed Central* PMCID: PMC3703013.

[59] Chan BS1, Sellors K, Chiew AL, Buckley NA. *Clin Toxicol* (Phila). 2015 Feb;53(2):131-3. doi: 10.3109/15563650.2014.998338. Epub 2015 Jan 19. Use of multi-dose activated charcoal in phenytoin toxicity secondary to genetic polymorphism.

[60] Howard CE1, Roberts RS, Ely DS, Moye RA. Use of multiple-dose activated charcoal in phenytoin toxicity. *Ann Pharmacother*. 1994 Feb;28(2):201-3.

[61] Mauro LS1, Mauro VF, Brown DL, Somani P. Enhancement of phenytoin elimination by multiple-dose activated charcoal. *Ann Emerg Med.* 1987 Oct;16(10):1132-5.

[62] Anseeuw K, Mowry JB, Burdmann EA, Ghannoum M, Hoffman RS, Gosselin S, et al. Extracorporeal treatment in phenytoin poisoning: Systematic review and recommendations from the EXTRIP (extracorporeal treatments in poisoning) workgroup. *Am J Kidney Dis.* 2015:pii: S0272-638601258-5.

[63] Asconapé JJ1. Use of antiepileptic drugs in hepatic and renal disease. *Handb Clin Neurol.* 2014;119:417-32. doi: 10.1016/B978-0-7020-4086-3.00027-8. PMID: 24365310 doi: 10.1016/B978-0-7020-4086-3.00027-8.

[64] Richens A. Clinical pharmacokinetics of phenytoin. *Clin Pharmacokinet.* 1979 May-Jun;4(3):153-69. PMID: 383353 doi: 10.2165/00003088-197904030-00001.

[65] Keller F, Maiga M, Neumayer HH, Lode H, Distler A. Pharmacokinetic effects of altered plasma protein binding of drugs in renal disease. *Eur J Drug Metab Pharmacokinet.* 1984 Jul-Sep;9(3):275-82. PMID: 6519129 doi: 10.1007/BF03189651.

[66] Konstantin G Gurevich. Effect of blood protein concentrations on drug-dosing regimes: practical guidance. *Theoretical Biology and Medical Modelling* 201310:20. https://doi.org/10.1186/1742-4682-10-20.

[67] Thorn Caroline F, Whirl-Carrillo Michelle, Leeder J Steven, Klein Teri E, and Altman Russ B. PharmGKB summary: phenytoin pathway. *Pharmacogenetics and genomics.* 2012. PMID: 22569204, PMCID: PMC3349446, doi: 10.1097/FPC.0b013e32834aeedb.

[68] Argikar Upendra A, Cloyd James C, Birnbaum Angela K, Leppik Ilo E, Conway Jeannine, Kshirsagar Smita, Oetting William S, Klein Erin C, Remmel Rory P. *Epilepsy research* (2006). PMID: 16815679. doi: 10.1016/j.eplepsyres.2006.05.015.

[69] Claesen M, Moustafa M A, Adline J, Vandervorst D, Poupaert J H. In *Drug metabolism and disposition: the biological fate of chemicals* (1982). PMID: 6130920.

[70] Fischer, J. H., Patel, T. V. & Fischer, P. A. Fosphenytoin: clinical pharmacokinetics and comparative advantages in the acute treatment of seizures. *Clin Pharmacokinet (*2003) 42: 33. PMID: 12489978.

[71] *Parenteral Dilantin® (Phenytoin Sodium Injection, USP) – FDA.* Available at: https://www.accessdata.fda.gov/drugsatfda_docs/label/2011/010151s036lbl.pdf. Accessed 25 June 2019.

[72] *Cerebyx (Fosphenytoin Sodium Injection) [prescribing information].* Pfizer Labs: New York. Revised March 2017. Available at: https://www.accessdata.fda.gov/drugsatfda_docs/label/2017/020450s003lbl.pdf. Accessed 25 June 2019.

[73] *Medscape – Phenytoin (Rx)*. Available at: https://reference.medscape.com/drug/dilantin-phenytek-phenytoin-343019. Accessed 25 June 2019.

[74] *Dilantin (phenytoin sodium) – FDA [prescribing information]*. Pfizer Labs: New York. Revised January 2009. Available at: https://www.accessdata.fda.gov/drugsatfda_docs/label/2009/084349s060lbl.pdf. Accessed 25 June 2019.

[75] *InfaTabs® Dilantin® (phenytoin chewable tablets), for oral use– FDA [prescribing information]*. Pfizer Labs: New York. Revised December 2016. Available at: https://www.accessdata.fda.gov/drugsatfda_docs/label/2017/084427s037lbl.pdf. Accessed 25 June 2019.

[76] *Dilantin-125 (Phenytoin Oral Suspension, USP)-FDA [prescribing information]*. Pfizer Labs: New York. Revised March 2014. Available at: https://www.accessdata.fda.gov/drugsatfda_docs/label/2009/008762s036lbl.pdf. Accessed 25 June 2019.

[77] Dean L. Codeine Therapy and CYP2D6 Genotype. 2012 Sep 20 [Updated 2017 Mar 16]. In: Pratt V, McLeod H, Rubinstein W, et al., editors. *Medical Genetics Summaries* [Internet]. Bethesda (MD): National Center for Biotechnology Information (US); 2012-. Available from: https://www.ncbi.nlm.nih.gov/books/NBK100662/.

In: The Pharmacological Guide to Phenytoin ISBN: 978-1-53616-980-5
Editor: Payal Sud 

*Chapter 4*

# PHARMACOKINETICS AND TOXICOKINETICS

***Vincent Lee[1,*], MD, MA and Melissa Tam[2], MD***

[1]Department of Emergency Medicine and Medical Toxicology, Long Island Jewish Medical Center, North Shore University Hospital, Manhasset, NY, US

[2]Department of Emergency Medicine, Long Island Jewish Medical Center, North Shore University Hospital, Manhasset, NY, US

## ABSTRACT

Phenytoin is a barbiturate derivative used primarily for its non-sedating anti-epileptic properties and commonly as a second line agent in status epilepticus. It is highly protein bound and its clinical effect is determined by the concentration of free unbound phenytoin. It demonstrates saturable nonlinear metabolism and has a narrow therapeutic index. Additionally, there is a wide inter-individual variability in clinical response to dosage that can be attributed to genetic variations in metabolism. These factors make it impossible to generalize dosing regimens. Patients on maintenance therapy with phenytoin must have their dosages individualized with monitoring of serum phenytoin concentration until a steady state can be established. While general ranges of a safe

* Corresponding Author's Email: vince.lee.86@gmail.com.

therapeutic serum concentration have been established from studies as early as the 1960s, understanding the pharmacokinetics of phenytoin may help underscore the importance of individualized drug monitoring and may aid in recognizing the multitude of factors that may lead to toxicity or under treatment. Fosphenytoin is a prodrug of phenytoin that was developed as a safer alternative to intravenous phenytoin but it has its own unique considerations and side effects will also be discussed.

## PHARMACOLOGY

Phenytoin (5,5-diphenylhydantoin) is an anticonvulsant commonly used for the treatment of epilepsy. It is available in both oral (as phenytoin or phenytoin sodium) and parenteral (phenytoin sodium) formulations. Phenytoin and phenytoin sodium appear as a white odorless powder. The melting point of phenytoin is 295-298°C. Phenytoin is insoluble in water whereas phenytoin sodium is soluble in water with a solubility of 1g/66mL and freely soluble in propylene glycol. Phenytoin formulations are available as tablets as 50mg tablets, 30- 100- and 125-mg/5mL oral suspensions. Phenytoin sodium formulations are available as 25-, 30-, 50-, 100- and 300-mg capsules, 30- and 100-mg prompt and extended release capsules, and 50- and 100-mg coated tablets [42].

Phenytoin's mechanism of action has not been well elucidated, but several hypotheses currently exist [10, 21]. It is unique in that it is able to suppress seizure activity without causing sedative effects at therapeutic levels [10]. This may be due to a preferential inhibition of high frequency neuronal excitatory transmission, allowing for normal neuronal lower frequency firing to proceed unhindered [21]. Additionally, phenytoin's effects on neuronal sodium, calcium, and potassium concentrations and alteration of sodium and calcium channel activity may stabilize the neuronal environment. By suppressing neuronal sodium action potential spikes, decreasing phosphorylation of calcium associated proteins (leading to more inactive calcium channels), and increasing intracellular calcium by inhibition of sodium/calcium exchange, phenytoin can decrease repetitive firing of neurons and the rate of neuronal after-discharges [21]. Furthermore, phenytoin demonstrates affinity for the benzodiazepine receptor site of chloride channels, likely enhancing gamma-aminobutyric acid (GABA) mediated neuronal inhibition [10, 21]. These proposed mechanisms of phenytoin do not explain its toxic effects as paradoxically, phenytoin at toxic levels may induce seizures, lethargy and symptoms of cerebellar dysfunction [9].

Phenytoin's anti-epileptic ability of inhibiting frequency-dependent sodium channels also accounts for its anti-arrhythmic effects. As a Vaughan-Williams class IB anti-arrhythmic, it was historically used during the 1950s-1970s to treat severe digoxin toxicity by improving AV conduction and reversing digitalis induced heart block [31, 34, 40]. By acting on sodium channels in cardiac myocytes, it decreases the rate of depolarization of the cardiac action potential and increases the effective refractory period. However, phenytoin has fallen out of use as an anti-arrhythmic in favor of the more effective Digoxin-specific antibody Fab fragment treatment [29].

## Bioavailability

Phenytoin is a weak acid (pKa = 8.06-8.3) [42] that is poorly water soluble. It precipitates in the acidic environment of the stomach and its bioavailability is largely determined by the size and surface area of the precipitant, which may vary based on the composition of the particular formulation or brand of the drug being used. Once dissolved, it is over 90% bound to plasma proteins in adults and 82-85% protein bound in neonates (mainly albumin and to a lesser degree to alpha-1-acid glycoprotein). It rapidly distributes in tissues with a volume of distribution of about 0.75L/kg in adults and 1.2 L/kg in infants and neonates [52]. The plasma concentration of serum phenytoin rapidly equilibrates within the brain tissue, offering rapid anti-epileptic properties when infused intravenously [16].

Phenytoin can be administered orally, parenterally, intravenously or intramuscularly. The parenteral formulation is a phenytoin sodium salt that contains 92% phenytoin by weight. Phenytoin may also come in capsules, tablets or suspensions of phenytoin sodium, and it is available in extended or immediate release formulations. Due to phenytoin's poor water solubility, the parental formulation must be delivered with a diluent consisting of 10% ethanol, 40% propylene glycol, and 50% water, with an alkaline pH of 12 [36].

Phenytoin may take as few as 1.5 to 3 hours or up to 22 hours once ingested in its oral form to reach peak plasma levels [16]. The large variability is secondary to co-administered medications that interfere with phenytoin absorption, the pH of gastric and intestinal contents that alters the amount of drug precipitation, and changes in gastric motility.

Additionally, phenytoin has been found to be a substrate of p-glycoprotein (ABCB1), a ubiquitous cell membrane ATP dependent efflux transporter, which contributes to decreased drug concentration when given by the oral route, and has been found to be upregulated in patients already on phenytoin [7]. Variations in p-glycoprotein expression at the blood brain barrier may further affect phenytoin CNS concentrations, contributing to phenytoin resistant seizures [7, 14, 17].

Bioavailability of phenytoin may differ based on the manufacturer as different formulations of phenytoin may affect the absorption of active drug and may have different dissolution rates. This is in part due to differences in the excipient (non-active stabilizing substance) of the particular formulation. In 1968, a phenytoin intoxication outbreak occurred in Australia due to a change in the formulation of phenytoin from a calcium sulfate excipient to a lactose excipient. The calcium sulfate had previously interfered with phenytoin solubility thus reducing phenytoin absorption. When patients were switched to the lactose formulation, a much higher amount of phenytoin was absorbed per dose, leading to cases of toxicity [65]. Since then, multiple studies have compared brands of phenytoin bioavailability and clinical equivalency with varying conclusions. In 1994, Rosenbaum et al. found 22–31% lower serum concentration of phenytoin with the generic formulation compared to the Dilantin brand formulation. In 1985, Kishore et al. evaluated the bioavailability of four brands of phenytoin available in the Indian market and concluded that total serum phenytoin levels and therapeutic efficacy did not differ significantly. In a more recent study by

Kinikar et al. a sample of 222 patients undergoing a brand to generic phenytoin interchange, resulted in equivalent rates of efficacy. Pre and post interchange seizures did not increase despite a lower phenytoin serum concentration in the post-exchange group. [3]. Thus, with the varying study results and case reports available, it is recommended that patients be assessed for adverse clinical response when drug brand interchange must occur [16, 61-65].

When phenytoin is administered intramuscularly, it exhibits slower absorption with longer times to peak plasma concentration. Due to its poor water solubility and weakly acidic properties, approximately 30% of the drug is immediately released while the remaining 70% precipitates, leading to erratic and delayed absorption. In the setting of better alternative medications, phenytoin's intramuscular use has almost been abandoned when intravenous access is not available [37].

When administered intravenously, phenytoin is rapidly absorbed but has been found to be associated with hypotension and arrhythmias. [11] These adverse effects have been found to be infusion rate dependent rather than dose dependent, and attributed to the cardiac depressive effects of the propylene glycol diluent formulation [11, 32].

## METABOLISM/ELIMINATION

Phenytoin undergoes enterohepatic circulation and is metabolized to the inactive compound 5-(p-hydroxyphenyl)-5-(phenylhydantoin) [p-HPPH] by hepatic cytochrome P450 enzymes, predominantly by enzymes CYP2C9 and CYP2C19. It is metabolized to diphenylhydantoic acid, catechol metabolites, and an arene oxide in smaller amounts. P-HPPH is then glucuronidated by uridine 5′-diphospho-glucuronosyltransferase and excreted in urine. Approximately 5% of phenytoin is excreted in the urine unchanged. Studies have demonstrated that changes in urinary pH do not play an effective role in mediating excretion [12]. Small amounts of phenytoin (5%) is excreted in feces and a small amount is excreted in milk [24].

It has been suggested that genetic polymorphisms of the CYP enzymes contribute to some of the inter-individual variability of phenytoin serum concentration. Genetic variations of CYP2C9 and to a lesser extent CYP2C19 affect the rate of phenytoin metabolism. A study by Kerb et al. investigated the influence of differing CYP2C9 alleles. It looked at a population of 96 of Turkish origin, and found that the increasing number of defective 2C9 alleles correlated with a decreased rate of phenytoin metabolism [5]. This is further supported by a recent review article summarizing 19 clinical studies and case reports by Franco et al. which came to a similar conclusion [4]. Animal studies have reported minimal influence of CYP2C19 enzymatic activity but this becomes upregulated when CYP2C9 enzymes become saturated. However, the clinical impact of this may be minimal. While genotyping prior to drug initiation is not routine, it can be a consideration for patients with abnormally high phenytoin serum levels.

Phenytoin dependence on CYP metabolism leads to many drug-drug interactions, which is a common consideration for patients who may be on several anti-epileptic medications. Concurrent dosing of phenytoin with anti- epileptics such as valproic acid, carbamazepine, phenobarbital and primidone, may lead to increased or decreased free phenytoin levels due to inhibition or induction of CYP enzymes and protein binding characteristics of the other drug, necessitating a thorough review of patients' medications. [See chapter 5].

## PHARMACOKINETICS

Phenytoin's narrow therapeutic index is well known and documented. In a recent study by Ku et al. a population pharmacokinetic (PK) model was implemented using electronic health record data to accurately determine a therapeutic index of 0.7-1.5. In some previous studies, the therapeutic index was approximately 2 [1, 53].

Initially, phenytoin demonstrates first order pharmacokinetics at therapeutic concentrations, as there is sufficient CYP2C9 enzyme for metabolism. However, as the CYP2C9 enzyme becomes saturated, it exhibits non-linear Michaelis-Menten pharmacokinetics (zero-order kinetics), that is incremental with high drug concentrations leading to its rapid accumulation [16, 24]. Phenytoin dosing must be carefully monitored. Due to its saturable metabolism, predicting drug half-life becomes individual and dose dependent. As the steady-state concentration increases, drug clearance decreases, leading to lengthening half-lives [16]. A study by Houghton and Richens demonstrated that the half-life may be as few as 13 hours at low phenytoin serum concentrations or as long as 46 hours at serum concentrations at the higher end of therapeutic range. As determination of time to reach a steady state is based on typical half-life, time to reach a steady state for phenytoin may vary from days to possibly weeks. Therefore, it would be inaccurate to check serum concentrations for a patient at a presumed time of steady state as they may continue to have increasing serum concentrations [16].

Confounding the metabolism of phenytoin further, there is wide inter-individual variability in clinical response to differing phenytoin serum concentrations. This is well exemplified in one study by Gannaway et al. wherein phenytoin dose was uptitrated at increments of 25 mg over months until symptoms of toxicity presented. Whereas some patients typically began exhibiting toxic symptoms such as nystagmus at 20 mcg/mL, in another individual toxicity was not reached at levels as high as 35 mcg/mL. Phenytoin serum concentrations were also found to fluctuate dramatically. One individual's serum concentration increased from 19 mcg/mL to 38 mcg/mL with one dosage increase and required a modified dose increase of every other day to tolerate the medication increase [2].

## MONITORING

Clinical studies have established that therapeutic concentrations of phenytoin are acceptable in the range of 10–20 mcg/mL and of free phenytoin to be in the range of 1–2 mcg/mL [16]. The pharmacologic effect of phenytoin is dependent on its free unbound form which is able to cross the blood brain barrier and mediate its anti-seizure effects. Several factors influence the concentration of free phenytoin including age, sex, comorbid conditions, presence of renal or liver disease, concurrent medications that may displace phenytoin from albumin, and hypoalbuminemia [see chapter 3]. Any factor that may increase the level of free phenytoin should be adjusted for as it may increase risk for toxicity [16].

Measurement of free phenytoin levels can be expensive and may not be readily available. Several equations have been proposed to predict a corrected plasma phenytoin level from measured plasma phenytoin concentration while accounting for factors such as albumin concentration. From this corrected phenytoin level, a free phenytoin level may be estimated as 10% of this number. The most widely used of these formulas is the Sheiner-Tozer (ST) equation initially developed in 1976 [20]. However, multiple studies have demonstrated a poor correlation with actual free phenytoin levels when patients have multiple comorbid conditions [see chapter 3]. In one small prospective observational study by Javadi et al. assessing neurocritical care patients, the conventional ST equation was only able to estimate the free phenytoin level with 66% accuracy [19]. In another retrospective cohort study by Parikh et al. evaluating the predictive value of three other commonly used formulas in intensive care patients, there was also a poor correlation [20]. These formulas may be more accurate when used in healthy patients with normal laboratory values. However, they may not need to be used for healthier patients as these patients may be better assessed on a clinical basis. These correction formulas are most useful for suspected cases of phenytoin toxicity where obtaining a free phenytoin level to confirm the diagnosis is not available. One example of its utility is apparent from a case report of a 69 year old male who had altered mental status, drowsiness and gait disturbance and who was on phenytoin for seizure prophylaxis in the setting of an intracranial malignancy. In this case, the patient's plasma concentration of phenytoin was measured to be 18 mcg/mL. The clinicians applied the Sheiner-Tozer equation and calculated a corrected phenytoin level of 27 mcg/mL, which is above the accepted therapeutic range of 10-20 mcg/mL. This patient's estimated free phenytoin level would be close to 2.7 mcg/mL. In this case, phenytoin was discontinued and symptoms resolved after stopping phenytoin by day two [35].

Another consideration in adequate phenytoin drug dosing is the requirement of dose adjustment due to obesity and sex. Obese patients (BMI >30 kg/m$^2$) will typically require larger doses as phenytoin has a significant volume of distribution (0.65-0.75L/kg). Accounting for this, a retrospective single- center cohort study was conducted assessing the role of obesity and sex on phenytoin serum concentrations following a loading dose. This study used a formula accounting for distribution of phenytoin into fat (derived from prior studies assessing serum concentration in obese patients) and determined a kg/mL loading dose and measured serum concentration of phenytoin as well as clinical effect. It demonstrated no variance in obese vs non- obese pts but did find that females had a decreased phenytoin concentration compared to males. Its conclusions suggested a minimal loading dose of 15mg/kg to reach adequate serum concentrations to confer clinical effect [13].

## TOXICOKINETICS

Phenytoin toxicity in patients may manifest as nystagmus, ataxia, lethargy and seizures. The earliest sign of toxicity has been found to be nystagmus but studies have demonstrated cognitive impairment that occurs even before the onset of nystagmus [12]. The most common presenting symptom in one retrospective observational study (n =30) was unsteady gait. In this study, four cases were due to iatrogenic intravenous phenytoin supplementation, while the remaining cases were oral overdoses (one intentional). Leading causes of phenytoin intoxication include prescription dosing misunderstandings, excessive self- medication by patients, drug interactions, and new dosing changes [11]. In a review of 4017 cases of phenytoin toxicity in the United States in 2002, 2103 were due to unintentional toxicity [6]. Patients who attempt suicide by taking a large amount of phenytoin may exhibit symptoms within hours. At 200 mg/day, time to clinical presentation of toxicity was found to vary between 1-3 days [11]. Phenytoin toxic effects are generally reversible if the cause is discovered early, however, it may result in death if toxicity continues unrecognized [11]. The lethal dose in adults is estimated to be 2 to 5 grams [66]. The lethal dose in pediatric patients is not known. Up to 25 times the therapeutic dose and serum concentrations over 100 mcg/mL has been reported to have resulted in complete recovery as reported by the Dilantin (phenytoin sodium) manufacturer package insert [66].

In a review of 85 patients on chronic phenytoin wherein levels were being checked, 20 cases of acute phenytoin poisoning was discovered. The clinical severity of symptoms was compared to plasma phenytoin levels. Of these 20 cases, 10 patients had disorientation and nystagmus at plasma concentrations between 20-30 mcg/mL, 6 patients had ataxia, nausea and vomiting at concentrations between 30-40 mcg/mL, and 4 patients had lethargy, confusion, bradycardia and arrhythmias with plasma concentrations > 40 mcg/ mL [44]. Other studies report observing drug-induced seizure activity at levels > 40 mcg/mL [36].

A review article assessing the frequency of serious clinical outcomes of phenytoin overdoses looked at 734 cases reported from 2000 to 2014. Data was gathered from the National Poison Data System and did not specify the acuity or method of delivery of phenytoin. Respiratory arrest was reported in 3.1%; respiratory depression, in 5.7%; coma in 16.1%; cardiac arrest in 3.5%; and 29 deaths. Other reported clinical signs of toxicity were seizures, lethargy, confusion, ataxia, nystagmus and hypotension [46].

Phenytoin is also associated with a wide range of adverse effects at nontoxic levels. It is associated with serious adverse hypersensitivity reactions including Stevens-Johnson syndrome, toxic epidermal necrolysis, thrombocytopenia, and anemia. When administered intravenously, it is associated with hypotension, arrhythmia induction, and local injection site pain and phlebitis. Its use during pregnancy is associated with teratogenic outcomes. Chronic use of phenytoin has been associated with hirsutism, gingival hyperplasia and cognitive dysfunction [6].

There is still much uncertainty regarding the mechanisms accounting for phenytoin's adverse and toxic effects despite over 80 years of research since the drug was released [10]. Some mechanisms are suggested to be due to the formation of toxic metabolites, such as in dermatologic hypersensitivity reactions, while others hypothesize that some reactions are due to idiosyncratic metabolism related effects. Some adverse effects are difficult to predict, whereas others are dose related and infusion related.

## CARDIOVASCULAR SIDE EFFECTS

Phenytoin is a Vaughan Williams class IB antiarrhythmic agent. Its antiarrhythmic effects are mediated by inhibition of cardiac voltage gated sodium channels, reducing the rate of depolarization of the cardiac action potential and increasing the effective refractory period [29, 54]. It also suppresses automaticity in ventricular muscle [55]. It was commonly used as an antiarrhythmic agent and in the treatment of cardiac manifestations of digitalis toxicity. In an early study by Bigger et al. assessing phenytoin's utility as an antiarrhythmic agent and its associated plasma levels, 70% of arrhythmias responding to phenytoin did so at plasma levels between 10 and 18 mcg/mL. This early study by Bigger et al. assessing 93 patients had two cases of adverse cardiovascular effect from phenytoin infusion. One patient demonstrated marked sinus slowing and profound hypotension, nausea and diaphoresis that resolved with cardiac pacing and did not recur at a subsequent reaction. The other patient was being treated for a high atrioventricular block and experienced complete atrioventricular block and cardiac arrest, with a peak plasma level of 22 mcg/mL [31]. These adverse effects indicated a need for cardiac monitoring during drug administration, but the cause was attributed to a vasovagal response or underlying cardiac dysfunction. It has since become known that intravenous administration of phenytoin can be associated with profound bradycardia, hypotension, asystole and cardiac arrest.

The cardiovascular adverse effects of parenteral phenytoin administration can be explained in part by the propylene glycol diluent used to maintain phenytoin in a soluble form. The depressive hemodynamic and cardiovascular effects of propylene glycol were demonstrated in a study using dogs. Propylene glycol was infused under controlled conditions and the subject's heart rates and blood pressures were monitored. At higher doses of propylene glycol, the heart rate was seen to decrease to a mean difference as great as 72.1 beats/min within 3-5 seconds of drug injection, with a similar reduction in mean arterial pressure and a marked reduction in sympathetic activity. The effects were transient with heart rate recovering to the level of the controls within a minute. The study found the mean arterial pressure similarly decreased and there was a marked reduction in sympathetic activity. Administration of atropine was able to halt these effects, suggesting that propylene glycol causes a vagal reflex that transiently decreases sympathetic activity [32].

The direct effects of phenytoin on cardiac conduction has been studied in animals and humans. Animal studies with rats and canines have demonstrated an inhibitory of effect of phenytoin on acetylcholine activity in the heart, and a depressant effect on the sinus pacemaker and atrioventricular conduction [34]. These associated effects may account for the cardiovascular depression seen with intravenous phenytoin administration. In a human study, the electrophysiological effects of intravenous phenytoin were studied in 14 subjects using his bundle recordings, evaluating atrioventricular conduction and atrial refractory period. This study found variable effects of phenytoin with almost equal number of subjects demonstrating atrioventricular node conduction shortening and lengthening, and little effect on atria refractory period. Phenytoin also shortened the QT interval [33].

The adverse cardiovascular and hemodynamic effects of intravenous phenytoin can be mitigated by slowing the infusion rate of drug. An acceptable safe rate of infusion has been determined to be 50 mg/min. A review article by Guldiken et al. looking at 32 clinical cases and 10 case reports where phenytoin was used to treat epilepsy or arrhythmia, found no death due to hypotension or bradycardia in 1,593 patients when the infusion rate was not more than 50 mg/min, though some infusion rates were adjusted when patients developed adverse effects. Elderly or those with comorbid cardiovascular disease had increased incidence of adverse events and poor outcomes. It is recommended that the infusion rate for these patients be slower and rates of 25 mg/min should be considered [40].

Oral phenytoin overdose has rarely been reported to cause adverse cardiovascular effects. A retrospective study by Wyte et al. evaluating 57 patients with oral phenytoin overdose, demonstated no clinically significant dysrhythmias during cardiac monitoring. Mean peak phenytoin levels in this study was 48.4 mcg/mL and there were no deaths reported. Similarly, a study by Curtis et al. looking at 94 cases of phenytoin toxicity, with serum phenytoin levels ranging from 21.4-90 mcg/mL, found no new electrocardiographic abnormalities associated with phenytoin toxicity and no cases of hemodynamic instability. All patients in this study improved with supportive care. This is further supported by another retrospective study by Evers et al. looking at 44 patients admitted for oral phenytoin overdose, with maximum serum phenytoin concentration of 75 mcg/mL, there were no circulatory complications, significant cardiovascular arrhythmias or deaths. The evidence suggests that in uncomplicated oral phenytoin overdose, routine cardiac monitoring may not be warranted [57-60].

Although there is overwhelming evidence that oral phenytoin overdose does not result in significant cardiovascular compromise, there exist case reports that suggest it is a rare but possible complication of phenytoin toxicity. One case report described cardiovascular toxicity with chronic phenytoin overdose resulting in a serum phenytoin level of 91 mcg/mL [56]. This patient was in a vegetative state and unable to demonstrate the early clinical signs of phenytoin toxicity-likely contributing to his continued overdose. He presented with hemodynamic instability secondary to severe bradycardia. Another case report described cardiovascular toxicity in chronic phenytoin overdose resulting in complete sinus arrest. This patient had a total serum phenytoin level of 36.4 mcg/mL [55].

## Infusion-Related Adverse Effects

Rarely, intravenous infusion of phenytoin leads to a phenomenon called ‘purple glove syndrome,’ characterized by a dusky discoloration of the extremity, blister formation, pain and loss of sensation. In one case study of a 26-year-old female, intravenous phenytoin was started for new seizures. Her symptoms started within a few hours of infusion and she was found to have thrombosis of the superficial dorsal, palmar and forearm veins. She recovered over the course of 2 weeks to a month, with splinting and pain control. The mechanism for this is attributed to the propylene glycol solvent and high alkaline pH of parenteral phenytoin, causing vessel damage and extravasation of medication, leading to surrounding vasoconstriction and thrombosis. However, there has been report of oral phenytoin being associated with purple glove syndrome [38].

## Hematologic Adverse Efects

### Megaloblastic Anemia

Phenytoin causes megaloblastic anemia because of the increased hepatic microsomal enzyme activity that is associated with its use [51]. This leads to increased use of folic acid, thereby depleting serum folate concentration, a vital cofactor in many metabolic pathways. Phenytoin is also structurally similar to folate and may interfere with folate transport due to this. Phenytoin’s alkaline formulation may also increase gastric pH, leading to decreased absorption of vitamin B12 (a weak acid that is better absorbed in an acidic environment) [51].

## IMMUNOLOGIC ADVERSE EFFECTS

Phenytoin use has been associated with a severe hypersensitivity reaction similar to drug reaction with eosinophilia and systemic symptoms (DRESS) syndrome. It is also called anticonvulsant hypersensitivity syndrome (AHS) due to the cross reactivity of this reaction amongst other aromatically structured anticonvulsants. It is a life-threatening reaction that can clinically present with varying severity of fevers, lymphadenopathy, skin eruption, renal dysfunction, hepatic dysfunction, and late myocarditis. It is estimated to occur in between 1 and 1000 and 1 in 10,000 exposures. Symptoms may not present until weeks after initial exposure, with a median time to onset between 21 to 28 days for phenytoin [48]. Several mechanisms of toxicity has been suggested to cause AHS including the accumulation of toxic phenytoin metabolites leading to impaired DNA repair, direct DNA damage, non-covalent binding of T immune cells causing an immune response, and impaired mitochondrial function leading to hepatotoxicity [47-49].

Phenytoin is rarely associated with idiosyncratic hepatotoxicity in some patients. The metabolism of phenytoin to para-hydroxyl-phenyl-metabolite leads to the formation of a reactive arene oxide metabolite that is detoxified by epoxide hydrolases. It is hypothesized that this intermediate is responsible for hepatotoxicity by altering mitochondrial function. In a study using rat models, activated metabolites of the anticonvulsants phenobarbital, phenytoin, and carbamazepine were formed and used to monitor the effects of these metabolites on mitochondria. It was found that these intermediate forms were able to decrease ATP synthesis, the respiratory control ratio (an indicator of mitochondrial coupling), membrane potential, calcium uptake/release and calcium induced swelling, and stage III and IV of the mitochondrial respiratory cycle. Phenytoin was determined to have the highest toxicity potential amongst the three anticonvulsants in the study [47].

Rarely, phenytoin hypersensitivity syndrome presents as a delayed pulmonary complication, several case reports describe bronchiolitis obliterans organizing pneumonia (BOOP) and cold agglutinin disease. This reaction can be managed with steroids, implying an immune mediated mechanism of toxicity [50].

# FOSPHENYTOIN

## Pharmacology

Fosphenytoin (5,5-diphenyl-3-[(phosphonooxy)methyl]-2,4- imidazolidinedione disodium salt) is a prodrug of phenytoin that was created in 1973. It was developed as a safer parenteral alternative to parental phenytoin. Approximately 75 mg of fosphenytoin sodium is equivalent to 50 mg of phenytoin sodium. Fosphenytoin concentration is usually expressed as phenytoin sodium equivalents (PE). It is water soluble with a solubility of 142 mg/mL. It is supplied in a ready mix solution in water buffered to a pH of 8.6-9.0 and is stable at room temperature for up to 48 hours [25].

## Mechanism

Fosphenytoin has no intrinsic pharmacologic activity but enacts its effects through conversion to phenytoin [16]. It is rapidly converted to phenytoin through hepatic enzymes with a conversion half-life between 8-15 min. The anticonvulsant properties of fosphenytoin are comparable to that of phenytoin. The mechanism of action involves modulation of voltage depending sodium channels, sodium/calcium exchange channels, and voltage dependent calcium channels, stabilizing the neuronal environment [43]. During its conversion to phenytoin, its hydrolysis releases inorganic phosphate and formaldehyde. Formaldehyde is converted to formate and does not accumulate in significant amounts [16, 37].

## Bioavailability

Fosphenytoin has complete bioavailability in either intramuscular (IM) or intravenous formulations. In contrast to phenytoin, it is soluble in aqueous solutions, has better tolerability when given intravenously and demonstrates better absorption when administered through the intramuscular route. When phenytoin is administered IM, it does not reabsorb in a predictable manner and may accumulate with deposits leading to erratic absorption. In contrast, fosphenytoin dosed intramuscularly will reach peak plasma concentrations within 30 minutes with a complete bioavailability. Dosing by this route has demonstrated similar plasma concentrations as that of oral phenytoin. It also offers a prolonged sustained release of medication at a lower dose as it redistributes from the tissue [37].

Fosphenytoin demonstrates higher protein binding than phenytoin (90-95% protein bound) and thus can displace phenytoin or be displaced from albumin in the same manner. This can be used advantageously by increasing fosphenytoin infusion rates to rapidly displace free phenytoin in the plasma, thereby obtaining a faster onset of clinical therapeutic effect. Infusion rates of fosphenytoin at 15-20 mg PE/Kg at 100 to 150 mg PE/min have been demonstrated to achieve similar phenytoin peak concentrations as that of parenteral phenytoin infused at 50mg/min [43, 25]. The conversion rate of fosphenytoin to phenytoin has been found to be shorter with a faster rate of clearance in patients with renal or hepatic disease [52]. This has been attributed to decreased protein binding and increased hepatic enzyme activity due to the respective disease state. Once converted to phenytoin, metabolism and predictive clinical response are similar to phenytoin.

## Safety

The safety of fosphenytoin compared to phenytoin has been explored in over 17 clinical studies with similar conclusions that fosphenytoin is as safe to use as phenytoin [66]. One double-blind randomized clinical trial in neurosurgical patients found comparable rates of adverse events between parenteral fosphenytoin and phenytoin sodium (32% and 39% respectively). This study also assessed the safety of intramuscular fosphenytoin. Of 118 patients who received intramuscular fosphenytoin, only 8.5% experienced adverse events. The most frequent adverse events in all groups consisted of central nervous system effects such as nystagmus, dizziness, ataxia, and somnolence [67].

Fosphenytoin has been demonstrated to be more tolerable than phenytoin. When compared, studies have demonstrated a greater degree of patient discomfort, pain and phlebitis with the use of parenteral phenytoin sodium versus fosphenytoin. However, paresthesia and pruritus occur more commonly with fosphenytoin, occurring at rates of 5-8% [27]. Though more rarely reported, fosphenytoin administration like phenytoin has been associated with purple glove syndrome. One detailed case report described an 81-year-old male receiving intravenous fosphenytoin for seizure control with a delayed presentation of purple glove syndrome. He first developed redness over the chest and arms, with his hands progressing to a painful purpuric discoloration. He had a phenytoin level of 25.8 mcg/mL at the start of these symptoms. He improved with steroids and as the drug levels weaned, he recovered. The mechanism of this phenomenon is still undetermined [45].

Fosphenytoin in comparison to phenytoin is less commonly associated with hypotension or arrhythmia, however, rare incidences of hypotension and bradyarrhythmias have occurred. A retrospective review of cases reported to the Food and Drug Administration's Adverse Event Reporting System databank found 29 relevant reports of adverse cardiac events related to the use of fosphenytoin between the years of 1997–2002. The cases reviewed included several high-grade atrioventricular blocks, transient bradycardia, and transient sinus arrest, necessitating temporary transvenous pacing in two cases [15]. Of the 29 cases, ten of these suffered cardiac deaths. The specific comorbidities of these cases were not specifically described but many had underlying cardiac disease, stroke, heart failure or infection, which may be confounding factors for the adverse cardiovascular events related to fosphenytoin use. However, these findings are consistent with other reports of fosphenytoin associated electrocardiogram changes and hypocalcemia.

One case report demonstrates that fosphenytoin may cause hypocalcemia, leading to associated electrocardiogram changes such as QT interval prolongation and ST interval prolongation. It is postulated in this case that when fosphenytoin is cleaved to release phenytoin, the inorganic phosphate that is released with it binds to calcium causing hypocalcemia. In this report, a 23-year-old male had normal calcium levels prior to a surgical procedure wherein fosphenytoin was administered. Electrocardiogram changes were noted within minutes of initiating fosphenytoin infusion during an operation. Despite slowing the infusion rate, the electrocardiogram changes persisted. Repeat serum testing obtained after the case demonstrated a therapeutic plasma phenytoin concentration but a decreased ionized calcium concentration of 4.52 mg/dL (reference range: 4.74-5.3 mg/dL) [39]. Hypocalcemia can lead to severe cardiovascular and hemodynamic compromise such as bradycardia, hypotension, heart block, heart failure, cardiac arrest and dangerous arrhythmias such as torsade de pointes [40, 41]. Cardiac monitoring should be considered when fosphenytoin is administered parenterally.

According to the manufacturer insert, the median lethal dose of fosphenytoin in mice and rats was found to be about 0.6 and 2 times the maximum human loading dose [43]. In a review article assessing the frequency of serious clinical outcomes of fosphenytoin toxicity from years 2000 to 2014, 208 total reports were retrieved. Of these cases, the majority of cases classified as serious (severe effects or death) presented with seizures (44%), hypotension (32%), bradycardia (24%), respiratory arrest (20%), and cardiac arrest (12%). These toxic outcomes are comparably fewer than that of phenytoin observed in the same study, wherein 734 cases were reported [46]. As fosphenytoin is a prodrug of phenytoin, its toxic neurologic manifestations are similar to that of phenytoin. According to its manufacturer insert, extrapolating from data of phenytoin toxicity, lateral gaze nystagmus can be expected at 20 mcg/mL, ataxia at 30 mcg/mL, and dysarthria and lethargy at phenytoin plasma concentrations over 40 mcg/mL [43].

## CONCLUSION

Phenytoin is an effective anticonvulsant drug that demonstrates multiple modes of action that has expanded its use to include treatment of a myriad of conditions affecting multiple organ systems, including atrial and ventricular arrhythmias, post-traumatic seizures, trigeminal neuralgia, chronic pain, wound healing. Although phenytoin toxicity rarely results in significant mortality, the symptoms of phenytoin toxicity such as nystagmus, malaise, headaches, lethargy, and ataxia are important for physicians to recognize as they may have subtle presentations. Due to phenytoin's narrow therapeutic index and wide inter-individual variability in metabolism, phenytoin serum levels should be checked until a steady state has been reached and then routine monitoring should be considered for patients who are on multiple medications or medical problems that may interfere with phenytoin metabolism. Physicians should recognize that phenytoin has demonstrated adverse effects across all organ systems. Although fosphenytoin offers a safer alternative to intravenous phenytoin, it has also been rarely associated with adverse cardiovascular effects and has a higher incidence of local adverse effects.

## REFERENCES

[1] Ku, Lawrence C., Huali Wu, Rachel G. Greenberg, Kevin D. Hill, Daniel Gonzalez, Christoph P. Hornik, Alysha Berezny, Jeffrey T. Guptill, Wenlei Jiang, Nan Zheng, Michael Cohen-Wolkowiez, and Chiara Melloni. "Use of Therapeutic Drug Monitoring, Electronic Health Record Data, and Pharmacokinetic Modeling to Determine the Therapeutic Index of Phenytoin and Lamotrigine." *Therapeutic Drug Monitoring* 38, no. 6 (2016): 728-37. doi: 10.1097/ftd.0000000000000354.

[2] Gannaway, Dj, and Ge Mawer. "Serum Phenytoin Concentration and Clinical Response in Patients with Epilepsy." *British Journal of Clinical Pharmacology* 12, no. 6 (1981): 833-39. doi: 10.1111/j.1365-2125.1981.tb01316.x.

[3] Kinikar, Shilpa A., Thomas Delate, C. Mindy Menaker-Wiener, and William H. Bentley. "Clinical Outcomes Associated with Brand-to-Generic Phenytoin Interchange." *Annals of Pharmacotherapy* 46, no. 5 (2012): 650-58. doi:10.1345/aph.1q601.

[4] Franco, Valentina, and Emilio Perucca. "CYP2C9 Polymorphisms and Phenytoin Metabolism: Implications for Adverse Effects." *Expert Opinion on Drug Metabolism & Toxicology* 11, no. 8 (2015): 1269-279. doi:10.1517/17425255.2015.1053463.

[5] Kerb, R., A. S. Aynacioglu, J. Brockmöller, R. Schlagenhaufer, S. Bauer, T. Szekeres, A. Hamwi, M. Fritzer-Szekeres, C. Baumgartner, H. Z. Öngen, P. Güzelbey, I. Roots, and U. Brinkmann. "The Predictive Value of MDR1, CYP2C9, and CYP2C19 Polymorphisms for Phenytoin Plasma Levels." *The Pharmacogenomics Journal 1,* no. 3 (2001): 204-10. doi:10.1038/sj.tpj.6500025.

[6] Craig, Simon. "Phenytoin Poisoning." *Neurocritical Care* 3, no. 2 (2005): 161-70. doi: 10.1385/ncc:3:2:161.

[7] Alvariza, Silvana, Pietro Fagiolino, Marta Vázquez, Iris Feria-Romero, and Sandra Orozco-Suárez. "Chronic Administration of Phenytoin Induces Efflux Transporter Overexpression in Rats." *Pharmacological Reports* 66, no. 6 (2014): 946-51. doi: 10.1016/ j.pharep.2014.06.007.

[8] Bergen, Donna C. "Pharmacokinetics of Phenytoin: Reminders and Discoveries." *Epilepsy Currents* 9, no. 4 (2009): 102-04. doi: 10. 1111/j.1535-7511.2009.01307.x.

[9] Al-Khulaif, Ali H., and Asaad S. Shujaa. "Phenytoin Induced Status Epilepticus." *Neurosciences* 15, no. 2 (2010): 131-32.

[10] Hesselink, Jan M. Keppel, and David J. Kopsky. "Phenytoin: 80 years Young, from Epilepsy to Breast Cancer, a Remarkable Molecule with Multiple Modes of Action." *Journal of Neurology* 264, no. 8 (2017): 1617-621. doi: 10.1007/s00415-017-8391-5.

[11] Hwang, Wen-Juh, and Jing-Jane Tsai. "Acute Phenytoin Intoxication: Causes, Symptoms, Misdiagnoses, and Outcomes." *The Kaohsiung Journal of Medical Sciences* 20, no. 12 (2004): 580-85. doi: 10.1016/s1607-551x(09)70262-1.

[12] Jensen, B. Nordentoft, and V. Grynderup. "Studies on the Metabolism of Phenytoin." *Epilepsia* 7, no. 3 (1966): 238-45. doi: 10.1111/j.1528-1157.1966.tb03802.x.

[13] Dasgupta, Ryan, Cesar Alaniz, and Danielle Burghardt. "Evaluation of Intravenous Phenytoin and Fosphenytoin Loading Doses: Influence of Obesity and Sex." *Annals of Pharmacotherapy* 53, no. 5 (2018): 458-63. doi: 10.1177/1060028018818785.

[14] Lai, Ming-Liang, Yu-En Tien, Ying-Syuan Huang, and Jin-Ding Huang. "Studies on Pharmacokinetic Mechanism of Phenytoin Resistance in Refractory Epilepsy." *Journal of Pharmaceutical Sciences* 102, no. 9 (2013): 3189-195. doi: 10.1002/jps.23593.

[15] Adams, Bruce D., Neil H. Buckley, James Y. Kim, and Lia B. Tipps. "Fosphenytoin May Cause Hemodynamically Unstable Bradydysrhythmias." *The Journal of Emergency Medicine* 30, no. 1 (2006): 75-79. doi: 10.1016/j.jemermed.2005.01.034.

[16] Richens, Alan. "Clinical Pharmacokinetics of Phenytoin." *Clinical Pharmacokinetics* 4, no. 3 (1979): 153-69. doi: 10.2165/00003088-197904030-00001.

[17] Thorn, Caroline F., Michelle Whirl-Carrillo, J. Steven Leeder, Teri E. Klein, and Russ B. Altman. "PharmGKB Summary." *Pharmacogenetics and Genomics* 22, no. 6 (2012): 466-70. doi: 10.1097/fpc.0b013e32834aeedb.

[18] Heine, Rob, Sean P. Kane, Alwin D.r. Huitema, Matthew D. Krasowski, and Erik M. Maarseveen. "Non-linear Protein Binding of Phenytoin in Clinical Practice - Development and Validation of a Mechanistic Prediction Model." *British Journal of Clinical Pharmacology,* 2019. doi:10.1111/bcp.14053.

[19] Javadi, Seyyede-Sareh, Reza Mahjub, Abbas Taher, Younes Mohammadi, and Maryam Mehrpooya. "Correlation between Measured and Calculated Free Phenytoin Serum Concentration in

Neurointensive Care Patients with Hypoalbuminemia." *Clinical Pharmacology: Advances and ApplicationsVolume* 10 (2018): 183-90. doi:10.2147/cpaa.s186322.

[20] Parikh, Labdhi, and Robert Maclaren. "The Predictive Performances of Equations Used to Estimate Unbound Phenytoin Concentrations in a Medical ICU Population and the Impact of Exogenous Albumin Administration." *Journal of Critical Care* 44 (2018): 95-100. doi:10.1016/j.jcrc.2017.10.028.

[21] Yaari, Yoel, Michael E. Selzer, and Jonathan H. Pincus. "Phenytoin: Mechanisms of Its Anticonvulsant Action." *Annals of Neurology* 20, no. 2 (1986): 171-84. doi:10.1002/ana.410200202.

[22] Kesselheim, Aaron S., Margaret R. Stedman, Ellen J. Bubrick, Joshua J. Gagne, Alexander S. Misono, Joy L. Lee, M. Alan Brookhart, Jerry Avorn, and William H. Shrank. "Seizure Outcomes Following the Use of Generic versus Brand-Name Antiepileptic Drugs." *Drugs* 70, no. 5 (2010): 605-21. doi: 10.2165/10898530-000000000-00000.

[23] Au Yeung SC, Ensom MH. Phenytoin and enteral feedings: Does evidence support an interaction? *Ann Pharmacother* 2000;34:896-905.

[24] Begum, Tahamina, and Faruque Reza. "Current Practice of Phenytoin - Revisited." *International Journal of Enhanced Research in Medicines & Dental Care* 3, no. 2 (February 2016).

[25] Boucher, Bradley A. "Fosphenytoin: A Novel Phenytoin Prodrug." *Pharmacotherapy* 16, no. 5 (September 1996): 777-91.

[26] Joseph, Mathew, Ananthp Abraham, Ajay Vidyasagar, Jayseelan Lakshmanan, and Shalini Nair. "Phenytoin Toxicity in Patients with Traumatic Brain Injury." *Neurology India* 62, no. 3 (2014): 285. doi:10.4103/0028-3886.136929.

[27] Kirschbaum, Karen, and Cheryle Gurk-Turner. "Phenytoin vs Fosphenytoin." *Baylor University Medical Center Proceedings* 12, no. 3 (1999): 168-72. doi:10.1080/08998280.1999.11930167.

[28] Musteata, Florin Marcel. "Clinical Utility of Free Drug Monitoring." *Therapeutic Drug Monitoring,* 2012, 75-101. doi:10.1016/b978-0-12-385467-4.00004-x.

[29] Wang, Louis W., Rajesh N. Subbiah, Michael J. Kilborn, and Richard F. Dunn. "Phenytoin: An Old but Effective Antiarrhythmic Agent for the Suppression of Ventricular Tachycardia." *The Medical Journal of Australia* 199, no. 3 (2013): 209-11. doi:10.5694/mja13.10224.

[30] Neuvonen, Pertti J. "Bioavailability of Phenytoin." *Clinical Pharmacokinetics* 4, no. 2 (April/May 1979): 91-103. doi: 10.2165/ 00003088-197904020-00002.

[31] Bigger, J. Thomas, Donald H. Schmidt, and Henn Kutt. "Relationship Between the Plasma Level of Diphenylhydantoin Sodium and Its Cardiac Antiarrhythmic Effects." *Circulation* 38, no. 2 (1968): 363-74. doi:10.1161/01.cir.38.2.363

[32] Al-Khudhairi, D., and J.g. Whitwam. "Autonomic Reflexes And The Cardiovascular Effects Of Propylene Glycol." *British Journal of Anaesthesia* 58, no. 8 (1986): 897-902. doi:10.1093/bja/58.8.897.

[33] Caracta, Anthony R., Anthony N. Damato, Mark E. Josephson, Michael A. Ricciutti, John J. Gallagher, and Sun H. Lau. "Electrophysiologic Properties of Diphenylhydantoin." *Circulation* 47, no. 6 (1973): 1234-241. doi:10.1161/01.cir.47.6.1234.

[34] Rosati, Robert A., James A. Alexander, Stephen F. School, and Andrew G. Wallace. "Influence of Diphenylhydantoin on Electrophysiological Properties of the Canine Heart." *Circulation Research* 21, no. 5 (1967): 757-65. doi: 10.1161/01.res.21.5.757.

[35] Imam, Syed Haider, Kristen Landry, Viren Kaul, Harvir Gambhir, Dinesh John, and Brian Kloss. "Free Phenytoin Toxicity." *The American Journal of Emergency Medicine* 32, no. 10 (2014). doi: 10. 1016/j.ajem.2014.03.036.

[36] Bauer, Larry A. Chapter 10. Phenytoin. *Applied Clinical Pharmacokinetics*. 2nd ed. New York: McGraw-Hill Medical, 2008. Accessed July 24, 2019.

[37] Stella, Valentino J. "Case Study: Fosphenytoin: A Prodrug of Phenytoin." *Prodrugs Biotechnology: Pharmaceutical Aspects, September* 1995, 1259-267. doi: 10.1007/978-0-387-49785-3_43.

[38] Santoshi, John A., Arockiaraj S.v. Justin, Jeeth I. Jacob, Samuel C.r. Pallapati, and Binu P. Thomas. "Purple Glove Syndrome: A Case

Report. Hand Surgeons and Physicians Be Aware." *Journal of Plastic, Reconstructive & Aesthetic Surgery* 63, no. 3 (2010). doi: 10.1016/j.bjps.2009.06.021.

[39] Keegan, Mark T., Lois R. Bondy, Joseph L. Blackshear, and William L. Lanier. "Hypocalcemia-like Electrocardiographic Changes After Administration of Intravenous Fosphenytoin." *Mayo Clinic Proceedings* 77, no. 6 (2002): 584-86. doi: 10.4065/77.6.584.

[40] Guldiken, B., J. Rémi, and Soheyl Noachtar. "Cardiovascular Adverse Effects of Phenytoin." *Journal of Neurology* 263, no. 5 (2015): 861-70. doi: 10.1007/s00415-015-7967-1.

[41] Akiyama, Toshio, John Batchelder, Jacob Worsman, H.weston Moses, and Michael Jedlinski. "Hypocalcemic Torsades De Pointes." *Journal of Electrocardiology* 22, no. 1 (1989): 89-92. doi: 10.1016/0022-0736(89)90026-5.

[42] "IARC Monographs on the Evaluation of Carcinogenic Risks to Humans: Volume 66." *Some Pharmaceutical Drugs* 66 (1996): 175-237. doi: 10.1016/0278-6915(91)90150-6.

[43] *Fosphenytoin Sodium Injection, USP Package insert*. Teva. 2007.

[44] Fernandez-Ibanez, A., R. Ugalde-Herra, J.a. Rodriguez-Getino, J.b. Garcia-Casas, and J.c. Diaz-Suarez. "Review of Phenytoin Poisonings and Their Analytical Characteristics." *Clinica Chimica Acta* 493 (2019). doi: 10.1016/j.cca.2019.03.1576.

[45] Newman, Joseph W., Joseph R. Blunck, Ronald K. Fields, and John E. Croom. "Fosphenytoin-induced Purple Glove Syndrome: A Case Report." *Clinical Neurology and Neurosurgery* 160 (2017): 50-53. doi: 10.1016/j.clineuro.2017.06.006.

[46] Anseeuw, Kurt, James B. Mowry, Emmanuel A. Burdmann, Marc Ghannoum, Robert S. Hoffman, Sophie Gosselin, Valery Lavergne, and Thomas D. Nolin. "Extracorporeal Treatment in Phenytoin Poisoning: Systematic Review and Recommendations from the EXTRIP (Extracorporeal Treatments in Poisoning) Workgroup." *American Journal of Kidney Diseases* 67, no. 2 (2016): 187-97. doi:10.1053/j.ajkd.2015.08.031.

[47] Santos, N.a.g., W.s.g. Medina, N.m. Martins, F.e. Mingatto, C. Curti, and A.c. Santos. "Aromatic Antiepileptic Drugs and Mitochondrial Toxicity: Effects on Mitochondria Isolated from Rat Liver." *Toxicology in Vitro* 22, no. 5 (2008): 1143-152. doi: 10.1016/j.tiv. 2008.03.004.

[48] Knowles, Sandra R., Norman Dewhurst, and Neil H. Shear. "Anticonvulsant Hypersensitivity Syndrome: An Update." *Expert Opinion on Drug Safety* 11, no. 5 (2012): 767-78. doi: 10.1517/ 14740338.2012.705828.

[49] Gallagher, E. P. "Effects of Phenytoin on Glutathione Status and Oxidative Stress Biomarker Gene MRNA Levels in Cultured Precision Human Liver Slices." *Toxicological Sciences* 59, no. 1 (2001): 118-26. doi: 10.1093/toxsci/59.1.118.

[50] Angle, Pamela, Peter Thomas, Brian Chiu, and John Freedman. "Bronchiolitis Obliterans With Organizing Pneumonia and Cold Agglutinin Disease Associated With Phenytoin Hypersensitivity Syndrome." *Chest* 112, no. 6 (1997): 1697-699. doi: 10.1378/chest. 112.6.1697.

[51] Hesdorffer, Charles S., and Dan L. Longo. "Drug-Induced Megaloblastic Anemia." *New England Journal of Medicine* 373, no. 17 (2015): 1649-658. doi: 10.1056/nejmra1508861.

[52] Browne, T. R., A. R. Kugler, and M. A. Eldon. "Pharmacology and Pharmacokinetics of Fosphenytoin." *Neurology* 46, no. Issue 6, Supplement 1 (1996). doi: 10.1212/wnl.46.6_suppl_1.3s.

[53] Greenberg, Rachel G., Chiara Melloni, Huali Wu, Daniel Gonzalez, Lawrence Ku, Kevin D. Hill, Christoph P. Hornik, Michael Cohen-Wolkowiez, and Jeffrey T. Guptill. "Therapeutic Index Estimation of Antiepileptic Drugs." *Clinical Neuropharmacology* 39, no. 5 (2016): 232-40. doi: 10.1097/wnf.0000000000000172.

[54] Ragsdale, D. S., J. C. Mcphee, T. Scheuer, and W. A. Catterall. "Common Molecular Determinants of Local Anesthetic, Antiarrhythmic, and Anticonvulsant Block of Voltage-gated Na Channels." *Proceedings of the National Academy of Sciences* 93, no. 17 (1996): 9270-275. doi: 10.1073/pnas.93.17.9270.

[55] Thimmisetty, Ravi K., Janardhana Rao Gorthi, and Mahmoud Abu Hazeem. "Oral Phenytoin Toxicity Causing Sinus Arrest: A Case Report." *Case Reports in Cardiology* 2014 (2014): 1-4. doi:10.1155/2014/851767.

[56] Lu, Cheng-Hsien, Chih-Min Su, Chia-Te Kung, and Yu-Chin Wang. "Life-threatening Cardiotoxicity Due to Chronic Oral Phenytoin Overdose." *Neurology India* 57, no. 2 (2009): 200. doi: 10.4103/0028-3886.51296.

[57] Wyawahare, Mukta, Pratheeshgeorge Mathen, Dharanipragadak Subrahmanyam, and Giridharan Srinivasan. "Life-threatening Bradyarrhythmia with Oral Phenytoin Overdose." *Journal of Pharmacology and Pharmacotherapeutics* 6, no. 3 (2015): 179. doi: 10.4103/0976-500x.162017.

[58] Wyte, Collette D., and William A. Berk. "Severe Oral Phenytoin Overdose Does Not Cause Cardiovascular Morbidity." *Annals of Emergency Medicine* 20, no. 5 (1991): 508-12. doi: 10.1016/s0196-0644(05)81604-x.

[59] Curtis DL, Piibe R, Ellenhorn MJ, Wasserberger J, Ordog G. Phenytoin toxicity: A review of 94 cases. *Vet Hum Toxicol.* 1989; 31:164–5.

[60] Evers, Martin L., Amir Izhar, and Arshad Aqil. "Cardiac Monitoring after Phenytoin Overdose." *Heart & Lung* 26, no. 4 (1997): 325-28. doi: 10.1016/s0147-9563(97)90090-x.

[61] Silva, Daniela Amaral, Raimar Löbenberg, and Neal Davies. "Are Excipients Inert? Phenytoin: A Follow-up Half a Century Later with New Insights." *Journal of Pharmacy & Pharmaceutical Sciences* 21, no. 1s (2018). doi: 10.18433/jpps29745.

[62] Gagne, Joshua J., Aaron S. Kesselheim, Niteesh K. Choudhry, Jennifer M. Polinski, David Hutchins, Olga S. Matlin, Troyen A. Brennan, Jerry Avorn, and William H. Shrank. "Comparative Effectiveness of Generic versus Brand-name Antiepileptic Medications." *Epilepsy & Behavior* 52 (2015): 14-18. doi: 10.1016/j.yebeh.2015.08.014.

[63] Kishore K, Jailakhani BL, Sharma JN, Ahuja GK. "Serum phenytoin levels with different brands." *Indian J Physiol Pharmacol* 30 (1986):171-6.

[64] Rosenbaum, David H., A. James Rowan, Linda Tuchman, and Jacqueline A. French. "Comparative Bioavailability of a Generic Phenytoin and Dilantin." *Epilepsia* 35, no. 3 (1994): 656-60. doi: 10.1111/j.1528-1157.1994.tb02487.x.

[65] Soryal, I., and A. Richens. "Bioavailability and Dissolution of Proprietary and Generic Formulations of Phenytoin." *Journal of Neurology, Neurosurgery & Psychiatry* 55, no. 8 (1992): 688-91. doi: 10.1136/jnnp.55.8.688.

[66] *Dilantin (Phenytoin sodium) 100 mg Extended Oral Capsule, USP Package insert*. Parke- Davis. 2009.

[67] Ramsay, R. E., and J. Detoledo. "Intravenous Administration of Fosphenytoin: Options for the Management of Seizures." *Neurology* 46, no. Issue 6, Supplement 1 (January 1996). https://doi.org/10.1212/wnl.46.6_suppl_1.17s.

[68] Boucher, Bradley A., Claudio A. Feler, J. Christine Dean, David D. Michie, Benjamin K. Tipton, Kenneth R. Smith Jr, Ronald E. Kramer, Byron Young, Bruce R. Parks Jr, and Alan R. Kugler. "The safety, tolerability, and pharmacokinetics of fosphenytoin after intramuscular and intravenous administration in neurosurgery patients." *Pharmacotherapy*. 16 no. 4. (Jul-Aug 1996): 638–645.

In: The Pharmacological Guide to Phenytoin ISBN: 978-1-53616-980-5
Editor: Payal Sud 

*Chapter 5*

# DRUG AND FOOD INTERACTIONS

***Jennifer R. Fiebert*, BCPS, BCGP, BC-ADM***
***and Allison Raich, BCPS***
Glen Cove Hospital, Northwell Health, Glen Cove, NY, US

## ABSTRACT

Phenytoin is an antiepileptic drug that displays complex pharmacokinetic characteristics. These unique characteristics result in clinically important interactions with other drugs as well as food and nutrients. In addition to being responsible for causing a significant number of drug interactions, phenytoin metabolism may also be adversely impacted by a large amount of drugs. The clinical implications of these interactions can place patients at increased risk for phenytoin toxicity and adverse events, or alternately may result in a subtherapeutic response which can precipitate seizures and result in drug therapy failure.

This chapter will review the mechanisms and consequences of phenytoin related drug-drug and drug-nutrient interactions.

* Corresponding Author's Email: jgreco2@northwell.edu.

## INTRODUCTION

The ability of a drug to reach systemic circulation and display activity is determined by numerous factors, including the route of administration, the rate of absorption, drug metabolism, distribution, and the speed of excretion. Concomitant administration of a medication with another drug, certain nutrients or even foods can lead to interactions that can alter any of these physiologic processes. Interactions have the potential to cause changes in serum concentrations of co-administered drugs, resulting in increased risk for toxicity or reduced therapeutic activity.

Interactions are generally pharmacokinetic or pharmacodynamic in nature. Pharmacokinetic interactions involve changes in drug absorption, distribution, metabolism or excretion which can result in altered serum concentration of the affected drug. Antiepileptic drugs such as phenytoin exhibit complicated pharmacokinetic properties which can precipitate significant drug interactions [2]. Pharmacodynamic interactions modify pharmacologic effects and involve synergism and antagonism at the site of action. Antiepileptic drug interactions with clinical significance most often result from induction or inhibition of drug metabolism [1].

The clinical significance of individual drug interactions is often difficult to quantify due to a variety of potential confounding factors. The degree of clinical importance of an interaction may be affected by drug doses and serum concentrations of each agent, comorbid disease states, and patient specific factors such as individualized genetics which impact the expression of enzymes involved in drug metabolism and pharmacodynamic sensitivity to drug effects [1].

# MECHANISMS OF INTERACTION

## Pharmacokinetic Interactions

### *Absorption*

Phenytoin displays poor water solubility and absorption is dependent on the specific formulation used as well as patient factors such as gastrointestinal motility, the presence of bile salts, and composition of coingested food [3]. Phenytoin is available in the acid or sodium salt form and dosage forms include intravenous injection, oral suspension, oral chewable tablets, capsules, and extended release capsules. Absorption time and time to peak concentrations differ depending on the individual characteristics of the product and dosage form (sodium salt or free acid, particle size and shape, fillers and excipients, disintegration time, and dissolution rate [3]. Overall, orally administered phenytoin results in good gastrointestinal absorption. However, several drug interactions can interfere with absorption. Antacids containing divalent cations, sucralfate, and enteral feeding formulas can markedly impair the absorption of phenytoin, resulting in decreased serum concentrations [2, 4, 5]. Coadministration with food has the potential to cause an interaction as food-induced alterations in absorption can significantly influence drug concentration [3, 4].

### *Distribution and Protein Binding*

Phenytoin is highly bound to serum proteins, notably albumin. For drugs that are highly protein bound, changes in protein binding may cause significant interactions and can complicate therapeutic drug monitoring. Serum drug levels often look at the total serum concentration, which includes both bound and unbound drug fractions. However, only the free (unbound) drug is pharmacologically active and able to cross the endothelium to reach target sites in the tissues. If a displacement interaction occurs, the total drug concentrations will underestimate the amount of unbound, pharmacologically active drug [1].

Drug interactions occur when two highly protein-bound drugs (>90% bound) are administered concurrently and compete for a limited number of binding sites [2]. Displacement of phenytoin from its plasma protein-binding site by another highly bound drug (such as valproic acid) can cause the free, pharmacologically active fraction to increase considerably [2]. The free drug is then available to interact with both pharmacologic receptors as well as hepatic drug metabolizing enzymes.

Phenytoin undergoes significant hepatic clearance. Since systemic clearance of phenytoin depends on the unbound concentration present in the liver, as the free fraction of drug increases so does total systemic clearance [2]. This leads to a reduction in the total measured drug concentration. Even though unbound drug concentrations may transiently increase after displacement at steady state, assuming that there has been no alteration in the drug-metabolizing enzyme activity, unbound concentrations should return to their baseline values [2].

Generally, even when displacement interactions occur, the amount of drug displaced is a small amount of the total drug in the serum [1]. Additionally, the displaced drug is eliminated more quickly. The overall outcome of protein binding interactions is a decrease in total serum concentration of the displaced drug without any significant change in the concentration of unbound, pharmacologically active drug [1]. In this setting, unbound or free serum drug monitoring should be performed.

In addition to phenytoin, antiepileptic drugs that are highly protein-bound include valproate and tiagabine [2]. Displacement can occur, but the clinical significance is unclear. Despite being highly protein bound, tiagabine does not displace either phenytoin or valproate [2]. If phenytoin and valproate are co-administered, a complex interaction can occur due to protein-binding displacement as well as inhibition of metabolism [2]. Naproxen sodium and aspirin have also been reported to displace drugs from their binding sites and could cause intermittent toxicity.

*Metabolism*

Many significant interactions with phenytoin occur due to interference with hepatic metabolism. Phenytoin is metabolized by the cytochrome P450

(CYP) enzymes CYP2C9, responsible for ~ 80% of its metabolism, and CYP2C19, which metabolizes the remaining 20% [6]. A drug that interacts with CYP2C9 (for example, amiodarone) will have a greater effect on the serum levels of phenytoin than a drug that interacts with CYP2C19 (for example, cimetidine) [6]. Numerous drugs as well as endogenous compounds (such as free fatty acids, prostaglandins, steroid hormones and vitamins), are also metabolized by CYP2C9 and CYP2C19, leading to interactions [2]. Phenytoin is primarily metabolized via CYP2C9 to an inactive metabolite, hydroxyphenytoin, 5-(4'-hydroxyphenyl)-5-phenylhydantoin or p-HPPH), then glucuronidated. Hydroxyphenytoin is glucuronidated by uridin-glucuronyl transferases (UGT), specifically UGT1A1, UGT1A4, UGT1A6 and UGT1A9 [7]. Phenytoin also displays saturable metabolism, which is another potential mechanism for drug interactions [6].

As phenytoin is a substrate of CYP2C9 and CYP2C19, drugs that inhibit these enzymes can cause increases in the serum concentration of phenytoin [8]. Additionally, phenytoin is considered a broad hepatic enzyme inducer affecting several cytochrome P450 systems. Pharmacogenomics may also impact phenytoin metabolism and the relevance of drug interactions.

*Enzyme Induction*

Phenytoin is a potent inducer of some cytochrome P450 enzyme pathways. Hepatic enzyme induction increases the synthesis of new enzymes and ultimately results in an increased metabolism of the affected drug, leading to a decrease in its serum concentrations and pharmacological effect [1]. Enzyme induction is a gradual, dose-dependent process that can occur over several days to weeks depending on the half-life of the inducing drug and the synthesis rate of the metabolizing enzyme [2]. Importantly, when an inducer is removed, the serum concentration of the affected drug will increase, possibly leading to adverse effects or toxicity [9].

If a drug is converted to an active or toxic metabolite, enzyme induction may increase the concentration of the active metabolite and lead to greater clinical activity. For example, the addition of phenytoin to carbamazepine may lower carbamazepine concentrations but increase concentrations of its active stable metabolite, carbamazepine epoxide [2].

Phenytoin is a broad-spectrum inducer of several cytochrome P450 enzymes, including CYP2C9, CYP2C19, CYP1A2 (weak), CYP2B6 (weak) and CYP3A4 (strong), as well as UGT 1A1 and P-glycoprotein and can cause a clinically significant increase in the clearance of other classes of drugs [6, 9, 10]. Interactions due to the induction activity of phenytoin result in reduced efficacy of coadministered medications such as oral anticoagulants, calcium antagonists, steroids, antimicrobial and antineoplastic drugs [1].

*Enzyme Inhibition*

Enzyme inhibition is the process by which a drug inhibits the activity of enzymes metabolizing other drugs. Enzyme inhibition typically occurs when two drugs compete for occupancy of the same enzyme site. If a significant amount of drug is prevented from occupying the targeted enzyme site, decreased metabolism and thus an increase in the serum concentration of the drug occurs [2]. As opposed to enzyme induction, enzyme inhibition typically occurs rapidly (immediately to within 24 hours), increasing in effect with increasing dose and concentration. Serum concentrations of the affected drug often increase very quickly, which can lead to acute toxicity [1, 2]

Phenytoin metabolism may be inhibited by many medications, including topiramate, oxcarbazepine, chloramphenicol, isoniazid, sulfonamides, the antifungals miconazole and fluconazole, ticlopidine, cimetidine, omeprazole, diltiazem, disulfiram, trazodone, fluoxetine, imipramine, metronidazole, and amiodarone [2]. The clinical effects of these interactions are highly variable, ranging from insignificant effects in some patients to severe toxicity in others. Genetic polymorphisms and the complex metabolism of phenytoin may account for this variability.

*Excretion*

Phenytoin is cleared primarily by hepatic metabolism (over 95%). Most of the drug is excreted in the bile as an inactive metabolite, which is then reabsorbed from the intestinal tract and ultimately excreted in the urine [7]. Renal elimination accounts for less than 5% of phenytoin elimination. Drug interactions affecting renal excretion are rare with phenytoin since only a small amount is excreted unchanged in the urine [6].

## Other Pharmacokinetic Mechanisms

### P-Glycoprotein (P-gp) and Other Transporter Proteins

P-glycoprotein (P-gp) is a plasma membrane protein which plays an important role in drug transport in many organs, including the brain. P-glycoprotein functions as a transmembrane efflux pump, pumping its substrates from inside to outside the cell [11]. The presence of P-gp can affect the absorption, distribution, metabolism and excretion of many drugs and over-expression of this protein can reportedly lead to subtherapeutic serum concentrations of some antiepileptic medications, including phenytoin which is a substrate for P-gp [12, 13, 15, 16, 17]. Similar to drug metabolizing enzymes, drugs which induce or inhibit P-glycoprotein can interact with other drugs handled by the pump, resulting in altered concentrations in the blood and brain [11, 14].

### Pharmacodynamic Interactions

Pharmacodynamic interactions occur when the action of a drug is altered by the presence of another drug. These interactions can result in enhanced activity (synergism) or decreased activity (antagonism) without changing the serum drug concentration. Interactions can occur directly at the site of drug action or indirectly by interfering with other physiologic mechanisms. As opposed to pharmacokinetic interactions, pharmacodynamic interactions are more difficult to identify and quantify.

# SPECIAL POPULATIONS

Certain patient populations or individuals may be more vulnerable to phenytoin related drug interactions.

## Genetic Polymorphism

Genetic mutations of the isoenzymes involved in drug metabolism may explain the variability in patient response to certain drugs or vulnerability to toxicity. Polymorphism among the cytochrome P450 family of hepatic enzymes occurs in varying degrees of frequency among different ethnicities [6]. Mutations of CYP2C9 or CYP2C19 results in impaired metabolism of several antiepileptic drugs, including phenytoin [6]. Polymorphism of the CYP2C9 gene occurs at a higher frequently in Caucasian patients than in Japanese or other Asian patient populations, whereas the frequency of mutations of the CYP2C19 gene is much higher in Japanese than in Caucasian patients [18].

Pharmacogenetic screening for patient CYP2C9 status may help guide phenytoin prescribing and identify patients at higher risk for adverse effects. For example, reducing the phenytoin starting dose by 50% may be reasonable in CYP2C9 poor metabolizers, whereby a 25% reduction in starting dose may be reasonable in CYP2C9 intermediate metabolizers [19]. Evaluating serum concentrations and clinical response after 7 to 10 days of therapy is recommended [20].

## Elderly Patients

Physiological changes that occur with aging result in alterations in pharmacokinetics and pharmacodynamics and affect how older patients respond to drug therapy. Choice of appropriate drug, dose, dosing frequency and monitoring must be carefully considered in the geriatric population. Older patients generally take a higher number of medications than younger patients and they are particularly vulnerable to drug-drug interactions. Geriatric patients are also more susceptible to the adverse effects of drug interactions due age related pharmacokinetic and pharmacodynamic changes.

Clinically, the most significant pharmacokinetic changes that occur with aging relate to renal elimination and metabolism of drugs. Renal function declines with aging, necessitating dosage adjustments for drugs that are renally eliminated [21]. Additionally, the ability of the liver to metabolize certain drugs also declines with age [21]. Pharmacodynamically, older patients are more sensitive to drugs that affect the central nervous system, such as phenytoin, and side effects of these agents are often exaggerated, leading to increased risk of toxicity [6]. Because of these changes, close monitoring of both therapeutic efficacy as well as adverse effects is necessary in older patients.

The pharmacokinetic changes that occur with aging that impact phenytoin specifically include changes in distribution and hepatic metabolism. In terms of drug distribution, serum albumin levels decrease with age, resulting in an increased free fraction of drugs highly bound to albumin such as phenytoin and increasing the risk of toxicity. Age-related reductions in hepatic clearance increase the bioavailability of certain drugs, including phenytoin. Phase I hepatic metabolism is decreased in the elderly, and drugs metabolized by phase I, including phenytoin, may need dose reduction or prolonged dosing intervals. Additionally, induction of CYP450 metabolism by certain drugs (including phenytoin) may be decreased in older adults. Overall, phenytoin clearance is decreased in geriatric patients and lower doses or less frequent dosing may be required.

# DRUG-DRUG PHARMCOKINETIC INTERACTIONS

## Antiepileptic Drugs

Many antiepileptic drugs have a narrow therapeutic index and also affect the activity of drug metabolizing enzymes. This leads to numerous clinically significant drug interactions which have the potential to cause adverse effects and toxicity [9, 22]. Phenytoin is associated with more drug interactions than any other antiepileptic medication due to its saturable metabolism, which is readily inhibited and induced [6, 23]. A slight inhibition of metabolism can lead to disproportionate increases in drug concentration and a risk of toxicity [6].

Several antiepileptic drugs are broad-spectrum inducers of CYP isoenzymes, as well as UGT. These include phenytoin, carbamazepine, primidone, and phenobarbital [2]. In general, the clearance of carbamazepine, phenytoin, primidone, valproate, topiramate, tiagabine, lamotrigine, and zonisamide is markedly increased by any of these enzyme inducers [2]. This can result in significantly increased dosage requirements of valproic acid, lamotrigine, and tiagabine in patients taking phenytoin [24].

Clinically important interactions that occur due to inhibition of phenytoin metabolism and thus increase phenytoin blood concentrations include: acetazolamide, clobazam, eslicarbazepine acetate, felbamate, methsuximide, oxcarbazepine, rufinamide, stiripentol, sulthiame, and topiramate [23, 25]. Table 5.2 lists additional drug interactions with antiepileptic agents.

**Table 5.1. Drug interactions by class**

| | |
|---|---|
| Antiepileptics | Table 5.2 |
| Antimicrobials/Antifungals | Table 5.3 |
| Antidepressants/Antipsychotics | Table 5.4 |
| Antineoplastics | Table 5.5 |
| Antiretrovirals | Table 5.6 |
| Anticoagulants/Antiplatelets | Table 5.7 |

CYP2C19 is a minor pathway of phenytoin metabolism but becomes more significant as the major pathway, CYP2C9, becomes saturated at higher phenytoin concentrations [2]. Oxcarbazepine, eslicarbazepine, and topiramate inhibit CYP2C19, causing a moderate increase (usually by < 50%) in phenytoin concentrations [1, 2, 6]. The topiramate/phenytoin interaction may become significant only at higher serum phenytoin concentrations [2]. Rufinamide may also increase slightly (usually by < 20%) serum phenytoin concentrations, but the mechanism of these interactions is unclear [1, 26].

## Valproic Acid

Valproic acid co-administered with phenytoin results in a complex drug interaction. Protein-binding displacement causes total phenytoin concentrations to decrease, but free concentrations increase because of the combined effects of displacement and enzyme inhibition [2]. Valproic acid inhibits the activity of UGT enzymes (UGT1A4 and UGT2B7) as well as CYP2C9, and, weakly, CYP2C19 and CYP3A4 and is considered a broad-spectrum enzyme inhibitor [1, 27]. Since valproic acid both weakly inhibits phenytoin metabolism as well as displaces phenytoin from albumin, the net result is that the free phenytoin concentration is unaffected despite the reduced total serum concentration [6]. In most cases, no dose adjustment is required. Adjustment of phenytoin dosing should be guided by based on free phenytoin measurement [6]. Occasionally, adding valproic acid to phenytoin may lead to elevation of both total and free phenytoin concentrations, increasing the risk of toxicity and requiring a decrease in phenytoin dose [1, 6].

# Table 5.2. Antiepileptic drug interactions

| Antiepileptics | Mechanism of Interaction | Clinical Effect |
|---|---|---|
| Carbamazepine | Phenytoin inhibits the metabolism of carbamazepine | Increased concentration of carbamazepine |
| Clobazam | Phenytoin induces the metabolism of clobazam<br>Clobazam may cause slight to moderate increases in phenytoin concentrations | Decreased concentrations of clobazam<br>Increased phenytoin concentrations |
| Diazepam | Phenytoin induces the metabolism of diazepam | Decreased diazepam concentration |
| Eslicarbazepine acetate | Phenytoin induces eslicarbazepine metabolism<br>Eslicarbazepine may inhibitor the metabolism of phenytoin | Decreased eslicarbazepine concentrations<br>Increased phenytoin concentrations |
| Ethosuxamide | Phenytoin enhances ethosuxamide elimination | Decreased ethosuximide concentration |
| Felbamate | Phenytoin enhances felbamate elimination<br>Felbamate inhibits phenytoin clearance | Decreased felbamate concentrations<br>Felbamate may cause marked increase in phenytoin concentrations |
| Lamotrigine | Phenytoin may increase metabolism of lamotrigine | Decreased concentration of lamotrigine |
| Oxcarbazepine | Phenytoin enhances the metabolism of oxcarbazepine | Decreased concentration of 10-hydroxycarbazepine |
| Phenobarbital | Phenytoin inhibits the metabolism of phenobarbital<br>Phenobarbital may induce or inhibit the metabolism of phenytoin | Increased phenobarbital concentrations<br>Phenytoin concentrations may be increased or decreased |
| Primidone | Phenytoin induces primidone metabolism<br>Primidone may induce or inhibit the metabolism of phenytoin | Decreased primidone concentrations<br>Phenytoin concentrations may be increased or decreased |
| Stiripentol | Phenytoin enhances stiripentol elimination | Decreased stiripentol concentrations |
| Tigabine | Phenytoin enhances tigabine elimination | Decreased tigabine concentration |
| Topiramate | Phenytoin enhances topiramate elimination<br>Topiramate may decrease the metabolism of phenytoin | Decreased concentration of topiramate<br>Topiramate may cause slight to moderate increases in phenytoin concentrations |
| Valproate | Phenytoin enhances valproate elimination<br>Valproate displaces phenytoin from protein binding sites | Decreased concentrations of valproate<br>Decreased total phenytoin concentrations, but free phenytoin may be unchanged or increased |
| Vigabatrin | Vigabatrin induces the metabolism of phenytoin | Decreased concentrations of phenytoin |
| Zonisamide | Phenytoin enhances zonisamide elimination | Decreased zonisamide concentration |

Source: References [1], [2], [6], [7], [23], [27].

## Non-Antiepileptic Drugs

Phenytoin interacts with many drugs in a wide variety of therapeutic classes. Drugs that interact with phenytoin that share the same mechanism as the valproic acid interaction include phenylbutazone, tolbutamide and amiodarone [6]. The inhibition of phenytoin is more pronounced with amiodarone, resulting in increased levels of both total and free phenytoin [6].

Drugs that inhibit phenytoin metabolism and increase blood concentrations include: allopurinol, amiodarone, azapropazone, capecitabine, chloramphenicol, chlorphenamine, cimetidine, clarithromycin, clinafloxacin, co-trimoxazole, dicoumarol, diltiazem, disulfiram, doxifluridine, efavirenz, fenyramidol, fluconazole, 5-fluorouracil, fluoxetine, fluvoxamine, imipramine, isoniazid, itraconazole, methaqualone, miconazole, nifedipine, nortriptyline, omeprazole, posaconazole, propoxyphene, risperidone, ritonavir, sulfadiazine, sulfaphenazole, sulfamethizole, sulfamethoxazole, sulfinpyrazone, tacrolimus, tamoxifen, ticlopidine, trazodone, verapamil, viloxazine, and voriconazole [23]. Drugs that induce phenytoin metabolism and decrease blood concentrations include: carboplatin, cisplatin, diazoxide, loxapine, nelfinavir, nevirapine, rifampicin, and theophylline [23].

## Acid Reducing Agents

Antacids such as aluminum hydroxide, calcium carbonate and magnesium trisilicate cause a rapid rise in gastric pH [6]. Generally, this decrease in stomach acidity does not result in clinically important drug interactions. However, antacids have been shown to slightly reduce serum phenytoin concentrations [6, 28]. In light of this finding, administration times of phenytoin and antacid preparations should be staggered in patients with low serum phenytoin levels to prevent absorption issues.

Proton-pump inhibitors such as omeprazole block the release of gastric acid from gastric parietal cells, resulting in increased gastric pH.

Omeprazole can increase plasma concentration of phenytoin by inhibiting cytochrome P450 CYP2C19, resulting in toxicity [6]. Plasma phenytoin levels should be monitored when these drugs are used together and also upon discontinuation of omeprazole therapy as omeprazole discontinuation without phenytoin dose adjustment can result in decreased phenytoin levels and increased risk of seizures [6]. Cimetidine, a histamine H2-receptor antagonist that rapidly reduces gastric acid secretion, is also an inhibitor of isoenzymes CYP2C19, CYP2D6, and CYP3A4, and can significantly interact with phenytoin [6]. Close monitoring of patients prescribed both agents is recommended, with a dose reduction of phenytoin typically needed [6].

## Antibiotics

Phenytoin can interact with several antibiotics, primarily through induction or inhibition of drug metabolism [1].

Phenytoin metabolism is inhibited by several antimicrobials. Isoniazid and chloramphenicol can increase the serum concentration of phenytoin and lead to possible toxicity. In contrast, rifampin induces phenytoin metabolism [1, 24]. Macrolides should not alter phenytoin. There are case reports of fluoroquinolones increasing phenytoin levels, but evidence points to interactions that result in decreased effects of phenytoin and increased risk of seizures with these agents. Ciprofloxacin has been reported to decrease phenytoin concentrations, though the mechanism is not fully understood [29].

Sulfamethoxazole-trimethoprim, a CYP2C9 inhibitor, can potentiate phenytoin toxicity by inhibiting the hepatic metabolism of phenytoin. Sulfamethoxazole-trimethoprim has been shown to increase the odds of phenytoin toxicity by more than twofold. When these drugs are used concurrently, monitoring for signs and symptoms of toxicity is warranted [29, 30]. Table 5.3 lists additional drug interactions with antimicrobial agents.

**Table 5.3. Antimicrobial and antifungal drug interactions**

| Antimicrobials/ Antifungals | Mechanism of Interaction | Clinical Effect |
|---|---|---|
| Cefazolin | Cefazolin decreases the protein binding of phenytoin | Increased free phenytoin concentrations |
| Chloramphenicol | Chloramphenicol inhibits the metabolism of phenytoin | Increased concentration of phenytoin |
| Ciprofloxacin | Ciprofloxacin diminishes the therapeutic effect of phenytoin | Decreased concentration of phenytoin |
| Clarithromycin | Phenytoin induces the metabolism of clarithromycin (CYP3A4) | Phenytoin can increase active metabolite of clarithromycin or decrease concentration of clarithromycin |
| Clindamycin | Phenytoin induces the metabolism of clindamycin (CYP3A4) | Decreased concentration of clindamycin |
| Doxycycline | Phenytoin induces the metabolism of doxycycline | Decreased concentration of doxycycline |
| Fluconazole | Phenytoin induces the metabolism of fluconazole (CYP3A4)<br>Fluconazole inhibits the metabolism of phenytoin (CYP2C9 and CYP2C19) | Decreased concentration of fluconazole<br>Increased concentration of phenytoin |
| Griseofulvin | Phenytoin induces the metabolism of griseofulvin | Decreased concentration of griseofulvin |
| Isoniazid | Isoniazid impairs the clearance of phenytoin | Increased concentration of phenytoin |
| Itraconazole | Phenytoin induces the metabolism of itraconazole (CYP3A4) | Decreased concentration of itraconazole |
| Ketoconazole | Phenytoin induces the metabolism of ketoconazole (CYP3A4) | Decreased concentration of ketoconazole |
| Levofloxacin | Ciprofloxacin diminishes therapeutic effect of phenytoin | Decreased concentration of phenytoin |
| Metronidazole | Metronidazole impairs the clearance of phenytoin | Decreased concentration of metronidazole |
| Moxifloxacin | Moxifloxacin diminishes therapeutic effect of phenytoin | Decreased concentration of phenytoin |
| Posaconazole | Phenytoin induces the metabolism of posaconazole | Decreased concentration of posaconazole |
| Rifampin | Rifampin induces the metabolism of phenytoin | Decreased concentration of phenytoin |
| Sulfamethoxazole/ Trimethoprim | Sulfamethoxazole/trimethoprim can inhibit the metabolism of phenytoin | Increased concentration of phenytoin |
| Voriconazole | Phenytoin induces the metabolism of voriconazole (CYP3A4) | Decreased voriconazole concentrations |

Source: References [1], [7], [23], [24], [29], [30], [31], [32], [33].

## Antifungals

Phenytoin interacts significantly with several antifungal medications. Fluconazole is an inhibitor of the cytochrome P450 isoenzymes CYP2C9 and CYP2C19 and can cause markedly elevated phenytoin plasma concentrations, often necessitating a reduction in phenytoin dose to minimize the risk of toxicity [6]. Phenytoin levels should be closely monitored when fluconazole is co-administered with phenytoin. No change in serum fluconazole levels occur when co-administered with phenytoin. Voriconazole is metabolized by CYP2C19, CYP2C9, and to a lesser extent by CYP3A4 [31]. Voriconazole interacts with phenytoin via phenytoin induction of CYP3A4 and results in significantly reduced voriconazole levels, which can be compensated for by increasing the voriconazole dose [31]. Additionally, administration of voriconazole, particularly in higher doses, can increase plasma levels of phenytoin. Phenytoin levels should be routinely monitored with dose adjustments as required when these drugs are co-administered [31]. Itraconazole is primarily metabolized via CYP3A4. Since phenytoin induces CYP3A4, serum itraconazole concentrations decrease dramatically, leading to itraconazole treatment failures [31]. It is generally not recommended for itraconazole to be administered with potent inducers of CYP3A4 such as phenytoin.

Posaconazole also interacts with phenytoin, most likely due to induction of UGT by phenytoin [33]. Reduced posaconazole concentrations are expected with phenytoin co-administration, potentially compromising antifungal efficacy. A reduction in phenytoin concentration can also occur in the presence of posaconazole, and monitoring of phenytoin levels is prudent [33]. Griseofulvin also interacts with phenytoin due to increased metabolism of griseofulvin resulting in reduced antifungal activity [1]. Table 5.3 lists additional drug interactions with antifungal agents.

## Antidepressants

Because of its enzyme-inducing properties, phenytoin stimulates the metabolism of many antidepressants.

Phenytoin's enzyme-inducing activity can decrease the serum concentration of tricyclic antidepressants (TCAs) such as amitriptyline, nortriptyline, imipramine, desipramine and doxepin primarily via CYP2C19 and CYP3A4 [1, 34]. This may lead to higher dose requirements of these antidepressants. Tricyclic antidepressants also have moderate to strong inhibitory potential on CYP2C19 and can interact significantly with phenytoin. TCAs, especially amitriptyline and imipramine, remarkably inhibit phenytoin metabolism and consequently increase the risk of phenytoin toxicity [35].

Phenytoin can also decrease the serum concentrations of mirtazepine via enzyme induction, possibly leading to increased mirtazapine dose requirements [36].

A modest decrease in paroxetine and sertraline concentrations occurs with phenytoin co-administration [1]. Additionally, sertraline can increase the serum concentration of phenytoin by decreasing phenytoin metabolism [37]. Fluoxetine can also inhibit the metabolism of phenytoin via CYP2C19, and levels should be monitored due to the increased risk for toxicity [1]. Trazodone can also increase serum phenytoin concentrations, potentially to a clinically important extent. Table 5.4 lists additional drug interactions with antidepressant agents.

**Table 5.4. Antidepressant and antipsychotic drug interactions**

| Antidepressants/ Antipsychotics | Mechanism of Interaction | Clinical Effect |
|---|---|---|
| Amitriptyline | Amitriptyline inhibits the metabolism of phenytoin metabolism (CYP2C19)<br>Phenytoin induces metabolism of amitriptyline | Increased phenytoin concentrations<br>Decreased amitriptyline concentrations |
| Clozapine | Phenytoin induces the metabolism of clozapine (CYP3A4 induction) | Decreased concentration of clozapine |
| Desipramine | Phenytoin induces metabolism of desipramine | Decreased desipramine concentrations |
| Doxepin | Phenytoin induces metabolism of doxepin | Decreased doxepin concentrations |
| Fluoxetine | Inhibitors phenytoin metabolism (CYP2C19) | Increased phenytoin concentrations |
| Haloperidol | Phenytoin induces the metabolism of haloperidol (CYP3A4 induction) | Decreased concentration of haloperidol |
| Imipramine | Imipramine inhibits the metabolism of phenytoin (CYP2C19)<br>Phenytoin induces metabolism of imipramine | Increased phenytoin concentrations<br>Decreased imipramine concentrations |
| Mirtazapine | Phenytoin induces mirtazapine metabolism | Decreased mirtazapine concentrations |
| Nortriptyline | Phenytoin induces metabolism of nortriptyline | Decreased nortriptyline concentrations |
| Quetiapine | Phenytoin induces the metabolism of quetiapine (CYP3A4 induction) | Decreased concentration of quetiapine |
| Sertraline | Sertraline inhibits phenytoin metabolism | Increased phenytoin concentrations |
| Trazodone | Mechanism unknown | Increased phenytoin concentrations<br>Decreased trazodone concentrations |

Source: [1], [6], [7], [23], [34], [35], [36], [37], [40], [41].

## Antineoplastics

Chemotherapeutic agents generally have a narrow therapeutic index with the potential for severe side effects. Any increase in drug activity that occurs due to a drug interaction can have massive effects on toxicity, while subtle reductions in activity can reduce efficacy and result in a suboptimal response.

Phenytoin can enhance the clearance of antineoplastics such as etoposide, cyclophosphamide and paclitaxel drugs by up to threefold [6]. The induction of cyclophosphamide and thiotepa metabolism by phenytoin can increase, to a clinically significant extent, the exposure to the active metabolites 4-hydroxy-cyclophosphamide and tepa, respectively, requiring a reduction in the dosage of both anticancer drugs [38].

Antineoplastic drugs that can induce phenytoin metabolism and decrease serum concentrations include vinblastine, cisplatin, bleomycin, and adriamycin (Vecht 2003). Table 5.5 lists additional drug interactions with antineoplastic agents.

## Antipsychotics

Interactions between phenytoin and antipsychotic drugs are common due to activity of cytochrome P450 enzymes.

Phenytoin can cause prominent reductions in the serum concentrations of quetiapine and clozapine due to inducing CYP3A4 [40, 41]. The metabolism of haloperidol is increased when combined with phenytoin due to phenytoin inducing CYP3A4, resulting in a reduced plasma concentration of haloperidol [6]. Table 5.4 lists additional drug interactions with antipsychotic agents.

## Table 5.5. Antineoplastic drug interactions

| Antineoplastics | Mechanism of Interaction | Clinical Effect |
|---|---|---|
| Abemaciclib | Phenytoin induces the metabolism of abemaciclib | Decreased abemaciclib concentration |
| Abiraterone | Phenytoin induces the metabolism of abiaterone | Decreased abiraterone concentraiton |
| Acalabrutinib | Phenytoin induces the metabolism of acalabrutinib | Decreased acalabrutinib concentration |
| Afatinib | Phenytoin enhances the elimination of afatinib | Decreased afatinib concentration |
| Alpelisib | Phenytoin induces the metabolism of alpelsib | Decreased alpelisib concentration |
| Axitinib | Phenytoin induces the metabolism of axitinib | Decreased axitinib concentration |
| Bortezomib | Phenytoin induces the metabolism of bortezomib | Decreased bortezomib concentration |
| Bosutinib | Phenytoin induces the metabolism of bosutinib | Decreased bosutinib concentration |
| Brentuximab | Phenytoin enhances the elimination of brentuximab | Decreased brentuximab concentration |
| Brigatinib | Phenytoin induces the metabolism of brigatinib | Decreased brigatinib concentration |
| Busulfan | Phenytoin induces the metabolism of busulfan | Decreased busulfan concentration |
| Cabozantinib | Phenytoin induces the metabolism of cabozantinib | Decreased phenytoin concentration |
| Capecitabine | Capecitabine inhibitis the metabolism of phenytoin | Increased phenytoin concentration |
| Ceritinib | Phenytoin induces the metabolism of ceritinib | Decreased ceritinib concentration |
| Cladrabine | Phenytoin enhances the clearance of cladrabine | Decreased cladrabine concentration |
| Cobimetinib | Phenytoin induces the metabolism of cobimetinib | Decreased cobimetinib concentration |
| Copanlisib | Phenytoin induces the metabolism of copanlisib | Decreased copanlisib concentration |
| Crizotinib | Phenytoin induces the metabolism of crizotinib | Decreased crizotinib concentration |
| Cyclophosphamide | Phenytoin induces the metabolism of cyclophosphamide | Increased concentration of cyclophosphamide's active metabolite |
| Dabrafenib | Phenytoin induces the metabolism of dabrafenib | Decreased dabrafenib concentration |
| Dasatinib | Phenytoin induces the metabolism of dasatinib | Decreased dasatinib concentration |
| Doxorubicin | Phenytoin induces the metabolism of doxorubicin | Decreased doxorubicin concentration |
| Duvelisib | Phenytoin induces the metabolism of duvesilib | Decreased duvelisib concentration |
| Encorafenib | Phenytoin induces the metabolism of encorafinib | Decreased encorafenib concentration |
| Enzalutamide | Enzalutamide induces the metabolism of phenytoin | Decreased phenytoin concentration |
| Erdafinib | Increased metabolism of erdafinib | Decreased erdafinib concentration |
| Erlotinib | Phenytoin induces the metabolism of erlotinib<br>Erlotinib inhibits the metabolism of phenytoin | Decreased erlotinib concentration<br>Increased phenytoin concentration |

| Antineoplastics | Mechanism of Interaction | Clinical Effect |
|---|---|---|
| Etoposide | Phenytoin induces the metabolism of etoposide | Decreased etoposide concentration |
| Floxuridine | Floxuridine inhibits the metabolism of phenytoin | Increased phenytoin concentration |
| Fluorouracil | Fluorouracil inhibits the metabolism of phenytoin | Increased phenytoin concentration |
| Fostamatinib | Phenytoin induces the metabolism of fostamatinib | Decreased fostamatinib concentration |
| Fotemustine | Phenytoin and fotemustine metabolism are induced | Decreased concentrations of phenytoin and fotemustine |
| Gefitinib | Phenytoin and gefitinib metabolism are induced | Decreased concentrations of phenytoin and gefitinib |
| Gliterinib | Phenytoin induces the metabolism of gliterinib | Decreased gliterinib concentration |
| Glasdegib | Phenytoin induces the metabolism of glasdegib | Decreased glasdegib concentration |
| Ibrutinib | Phenytoin induces the metabolism of ibrutinib | Decreased ibrutinib concentration |
| Idelasib | Phenytoin induces the metabolism of idelasib | Decreased idelasib concentration |
| Ifosfamide | Phenytoin induces the metabolism of ifosfamide | Decreased ifosfamide concentration |
| Imatinib | Phenytoin induces the metabolism of imatinib | Decreased imatinib concentration |
| Irinotecan | Phenytoin induces the metabolism of irinotecan | Decreased or increased irinotecan active metabolite concentration |
| Ivosidenib | Phenytoin induces the metabolism of ivosidenib | Decreased ivoidenib concentration |
| Ixabepilone | Phenytoin induces the metabolism of ixabepilone | Decreased ixabepilone concentration |
| Ixazomib | Phenytoin induces the metabolism of ixazomib | Decreased ixazomib concentration |
| Lapatinib | Phenytoin induces the metabolism of lapatinib | Decreased lapatinib concentration |
| Larotrectinib | Phenytoin induces the metabolism of larotrectinib | Decreased larotrectinib concentration |
| Loratinib | Phenytoin induces the metabolism of lortinib | Decreased loratinib concentration |
| Methotrexate | Methotrexate induces the metabolism of phenytoin<br>Phenytoin inhibits the metabolism of methotrexate | Decreased phenytoin concentration<br>Increased methotrexate concentration |
| Midostaurin | Phenytoin induces the metabolism of midostaurin | Decreased midostaurin concentration |
| Neratinib | Phenytoin induces the metabolism of neratinib | Decreased neratinib concentration |
| Nilotinib | Phenytoin induces the metabolism of nilotinib | Decreased nilotinib concentration |
| Nintedenib | Phenytoin induces the metabolism of nintedenib | Decreased nintedenib concentration |
| Olaparib | Phenytoin induces the metabolism of olaparib | Decreased olapraib concentration |
| Osmertinib | Phenytoin induces the metabolism of osmetinib | Decreased osmetinib concentration |
| Paclitaxel | Phenytoin induces the metabolism of paclitaxel | Decreased paclitaxel concentration |
| Palbociclib | Phenytoin induces the metabolism of palbociclib | Decreased palbociclib concentration |
| Panobinostat | Phenytoin induces the metabolism of panobinostat | Decreased panobinostat concentration |

## Table 5.5. (Continued)

| Antineoplastics | Mechanism of Interaction | Clinical Effect |
|---|---|---|
| Platinum derivatives | Phenytoin induces the metabolism of platniums | Decreased platinum concentration |
| Polatuzumab | Phenytoin induces the metabolism of polatuzumab | Decreased polatuzumab concentration |
| Ponatinib | Phenytoin induces the metabolism of ponatinib | Decreased ponatinib concentration |
| Radotinib | Phenytoin induces the metabolism of radotinib | Decreased radotinib concentration |
| Regorafinib | Phenytoin induces the metabolism of regorafinib | Decreased regorafenib concentration |
| Ribociclib | Phenytoin induces the metabolism of ribociclib | Decreased ribociclib concentration |
| Romidespin | Phenytoin induces the metabolism of romidespin | Decreased romidespin concentration |
| Ruxolitanib | Phenytoin induces the metabolism of ruxolitanib | Decreased ruxolitanib concentration |
| Sonidegib | Phenytoin induces the metabolism of sonidegib | Decreased sonidegib concentration |
| Sorafenib | Phenytoin induces the metabolism of sorafenib | Decreased sorafenib concentration |
| Sunitinib | Phenytoin induces the metabolism of sunitinib | Decreased sunitinib concentration |
| Teniposide | Phenytoin induces the metabolism of teniposide | Decreased teniposide concentration |
| Thiotepa | Phenytoin induces the metabolism of thiotepa | Increased active metabolite of thiotepa |
| Topotecan | Phenytoin induces the metabolism of topotecan | Decreased topotecan concentration |
| Toremifene | Phenytoin induces the metabolism of toremifene | Decreased toremifene concentration |
| Trabectidin | Phenytoin induces the metabolism of trabectidin | Decreased trabectidin concentration |
| Vandetanib | Phenytoin induces the metabolism of vandetanib | Decreased vandetanib concentration |
| Vemurafenib | Phenytoin induces the metabolism of vermurafenib | Decreased vemurafenib concentration |
| Venetoclax | Phenytoin induces the metabolism of venetoclax | Decreased venetoclax concentration |
| Vincristine | Phenytoin induces the metabolism of vincristine | Decreased vincristine concentration |
| Vindesine | Vindesine induces the metabolism of phenytoin | Decreased phenytoin concentration |
| Vinflunine | Phenytoin induces the metabolism of vinflunine | Decreased vinflunine concentration |

Source: References [6], [7], [38], [39].

## Antiretrovirals

Seizures occur more frequently in patients with human immunodeficiency virus (HIV) compared to the general population (~11% vs 2% respectively) [6]. Coadministration of antiretroviral agents and antiepileptic drugs is common in HIV-infected patients, and these agents can interact in significant ways. Many agents, such as lopinavir, nevirapine, indinavir, ritonavir, and saquinavir, are metabolized by CYP3A4, which is readily induced by phenytoin [6]. This interaction leads to subtherapeutic plasma concentrations of the antiretroviral agent, increasing viral replication and possibly the development of resistance. The dose of the antiviral drug may need to be increased [6]. Table 5.6 lists additional drug interactions with antiretroviral agents.

**Table 5.6. Antioretroviral drug interactions**

| Antiretrovirals | Mechanism of Interaction | Clinical Effect |
|---|---|---|
| Dasabuvir | Phenytoin induces the metabolism of dasabuvir (CYP3A4) | Decreased concentration of dasabuvir |
| Dolutegravir | Phenytoin induces the metabolism of dolutegravir (CYP3A4) | Decreased concentration of dolutegravir |
| Ledipasvir | Phenytoin enhances the elimination of ledipasvir (P-gp) | Decreased concentration of ledipasvir |
| Nelfinavir | Phenytoin induces the metabolism of nelfinavir (CYP3A4) | Decreased concentration of nelfinavir |
| Ritonavir | Phenytoin induces the metabolism of ritonavir | Decreased concentration of ritonavir |
| Sofosbuvir | Phenytoin enhances the elimination of sofosbuvir (P-gp) | Decreased concentration of sofosbuvir |

Source: References [6], [7]

## Oral Contraceptives

Oral contraceptive agents are very susceptible to enzyme induction. Loss of contraceptive activity can occur when these agents are used in combination with CYP3A4 enzyme inducing drugs such as phenytoin, which accelerates the hepatic metabolism of oral contraceptives [1]. The resulting potential reduction in contraceptive efficacy is particularly observed with low-dose estrogen oral contraceptives [6]. It may be necessary to increase the dose of estrogen when oral contraceptives are used concomitant with enzyme-inducing antiepileptic drugs to reduce the risk of unwanted pregnancy [6].

## Anticoagulants

### *Warfarin*

The effect of phenytoin on the anticoagulant activity of warfarin is difficult to predict. The addition of phenytoin to warfarin can cause a transient increased risk of bleeding when starting phenytoin, but a decreased anticoagulant effect during continued warfarin therapy [42, 43]. The exact mechanism of these contrasting interactions is unclear. Phenytoin may cause an initial displacement of warfarin from protein binding sites, resulting in an initial increase in warfarin effect [42]. With longer concurrent use, the decrease in warfarin effect may be due to phenytoin induction of CYP isoenzymes involved in warfarin metabolism [43]. In patients on anticoagulant therapy with warfarin, the INR should be monitored closely during the two to three-week interval following the addition or deletion of phenytoin therapy.

Additionally, warfarin may inhibit CYP2C9-mediated phenytoin metabolism, increasing the risk of phenytoin toxicity [42, 43].

### *Direct Oral Anticoagulants (DOACs)*

Direct Oral Anticoagulants (*DOACs*) include the direct thrombin inhibitor dabigatran etexilate and the factor Xa inhibitors, rivaroxaban, apixaban and edoxaban. Phenytoin interacts significantly with these drugs. Phenytoin can decrease the effects of the DOAC agents by inducing p-glycoprotein [44]. Additionally, phenytoin can induce the metabolism of rivaroxaban and apixaban via CYP3A4, decreasing concentrations of these anticoagulants [44]. Use of phenytoin should be preferably avoided in patients taking these anticoagulants as antithrombotic efficacy may be reduced. Table 5.7 lists drug interactions with anticoagulant and antiplatelet agents.

**Table 5.7. Anticoagulant and antiplatelet drug interactions**

| Anticoagulants/ Antiplatelets | Mechanism of Interaction | Clinical Effect |
|---|---|---|
| Apixaban | Phenytoin induces metabolism of apixaban (CYP3A4 induction) | Decreased concentration of apixaban |
| Aspirin | Aspirin can displace phenytoin from protein binding sites | May increase concentration of phenytoin |
| Dabigatran | Phenytoin enhances the elimination of dabigatran (P-gp induction) | Decreased concentration of dabigatran |
| Edoxaban | Phenytoin enhances the elimination of edoxaban (P-gp induction) | Decreased concentration of edoxaban |
| Rivaroxaban | Phenytoin induces the metabolism of rivaroxaban (CYP3A4 induction) | Decreased concentration of rivaroxaban |
| Ticagrelor | Phenytoin induces the metabolism of ticagrelor (CYP3A4 induction) | Decreased concentration of ticagrelor |
| Warfarin | Phenytoin induces the metabolism of warfarin<br>Displacement of either drug from protein binding sites may occur | Changes in concentrations of either drug may occur |

Source: References [7], [42], [43], [44].

## Supplements and Food Interactions

### Food

Phenytoin is a weak acid with limited water solubility. The time to reach peak concentration depends on both the individual formulation used as well as the dose. Due to phenytoin's narrow therapeutic window and nonlinear pharmacokinetics, food-induced alterations in absorption may have an impact on drug concentrations [3]. Food increases both the rate and extent of absorption of oral phenytoin and can impact its oral bioavailability [45]. Peak phenytoin concentrations have been shown to be significantly higher (mean increase of 40%) when the drug is taken with food than in a fasting state [45].

Even though food affects the rate of absorption, this is not likely to have a significant clinical effect because the relatively long elimination times limit the extent of fluctuation in serum concentrations [3]. However, a significant decrease in the extent of absorption could produce significant changes in phenytoin concentrations [3]. Accordingly, it is recommended that phenytoin should always be on a regular schedule with respect to meals. It is also recommended in an effort to prevent unintended changes in drug concentration that if a patient is stable on a certain formulation of phenytoin, the product should not be switched or changed unless there is a compelling reason to do so [3].

## Vitamin D

Vitamin D has many physiological roles within the body, including the promotion of calcium absorption. Long term phenytoin therapy can adversely affect vitamin D metabolism and bone health [46]. Through induction of vitamin D metabolism, phenytoin can decrease the amount of calcium absorbed from the diet and increase osteoporosis risk [2, 47]. Vitamin D status should be monitored in patients on chronic phenytoin therapy.

## Vitamin K

*Phenytoin* induces *vitamin K* metabolism, which can cause a relative *vitamin K* deficiency. Clinically, this is of significance in pregnancy, in which low levels of vitamin K may lead to peripartum bleeding problems in the mother or neonate [2]. In the setting of phenytoin use in pregnancy, it is recommended to supplement with 10 to 20 mg of vitamin K orally daily starting at 36 weeks gestation and 1 mg given IM or IV to the newborn [48, 49].

## Enteral Feeds

Enteral or parenteral nutrition can be used as an alternative feeding method in patients with inadequate oral intake. In patients with a functioning gastrointestinal tract, enteral nutrition administered through a feeding tube is the preferred method of nutrition support. A significant interaction between phenytoin and enteral feeding formula occurs when the two are administered concurrently [50]. When administered with enteral feeds, phenytoin absorption may be reduced by up to 70%, decreasing serum phenytoin concentrations to potential subtherapeutic levels [50]. The mechanism behind this interaction is not clearly defined, and it is unknown whether certain components of the enteral nutrition are responsible or if the interactions differ with different formulas (although higher protein feeding formulas have demonstrated a greater level of binding and less phenytoin recovery) [50].

One suggested mechanism is that phenytoin can adhere to the plastic tubing itself, resulting in impaired absorption [51]. Another potential mechanism is a physical incompatibility with the enteral nutrition, resulting in decreased absorption of phenytoin due to binding to certain components of the enteral formulations [51]. There is currently no standard approach to managing the enteral feed interaction, but several strategies can be implemented to maintain therapeutic phenytoin levels when enteral nutrition is necessary.

Staggering the administration of phenytoin is suggested to separate it as much as possible from tube feeds. Ideally, the feeds should be held for 1–2 hours before and after each phenytoin dose and the tube should be flushed adequately after drug administration [52, 53]. Immediate release phenytoin is administered multiple times daily, and holding feeds is logistically easier with bolus feeding as holding continuous tube feeds multiple times a day may result in a rate of feeding the patient cannot tolerate. To minimize the amount of time that feedings are held, phenytoin suspension should be given twice daily if possible [50].

If the enteral feedings can't be held, increasing the phenytoin dose is typically necessary to reach therapeutic levels. Even when phenytoin is separated from tube feeds, the dose of the phenytoin will still likely need to be increased to account for the interaction. Close monitoring of phenytoin levels is required to determine a therapeutic dose. For patients on a stable oral or intravenous phenytoin dose, the dose can be increased empirically by 50% when enteral nutrition is introduced [54]. Measuring free phenytoin levels to guide dosing is preferred, as patients requiring enteral nutrition typically have some degree of malnutrition and hypoalbuminemia may alter protein binding with phenytoin [54]. When enteral feeds are discontinued, a phenytoin dose reduction is usually necessary

The type of phenytoin formulation to be used with tube feeds needs to be considered. Patients taking extended release capsules once daily are typically converted to immediate release phenytoin, which is available as a suspension or chewable tablets. The suspension formulation can be administered through the feeding tube, and is available in both bulk bottles as well as unit dose. If the bulk suspension product is used, the bottle must be vigorously shaken and the dose administered immediately so the drug is evenly distributed in the suspension. If this is not done, the drug concentration may be higher in the bottom of the bottle versus the top, which could lead to inconsistent drug levels [53, 54]. Generally, chewable tablets are preferred over the bulk phenytoin suspension for a more consistent and uniform dose. However, in regards to enteral feeds, crushed tablets are more likely than the suspension to clog small bore tubes [54]. When phenytoin suspension is given through a feeding tube, it should be diluted with 20–60 mL of water to enhance absorption and increase the dissolution rate [50].

Other phenytoin formulations have been administered with enteral nutrition. Though controversial, opening phenytoin extended-release capsules has been utilized as a dosing strategy. A slurry of the contents of extended-release phenytoin capsules mixed with water and administered once daily with continuous tube feeding can be a dosing option [53]. Theoretically, if the micro crystal particles are not crushed when making the slurry, the extended release properties should be maintained enough to administer phenytoin once daily [54]. The tube feeds should be held for 2 hours before and after administration of the slurry formulation [50].

Crushing phenytoin chewable tablets is another possible dosing strategy [50]. Lastly, the parenteral formulation of phenytoin can be administered through the enteral tube, but it must be diluted because of extreme hypertonicity [50].

Whatever dosing strategy is used to minimize the phenytoin and enteral feed interaction should be maintained consistently throughout therapy with close monitoring of serum phenytoin concentrations and patient clinical response [50]. Consideration should be given to the type of EN formulation administered concurrently with phenytoin. If maintaining therapeutic phenytoin levels is problematic after employing the above strategies, intravenous phenytoin or fosphenytoin may be reasonable alternatives until the patient can tolerate oral medications [54].

## Folic Acid

Decreased levels of folic acid can occur in patients receiving long term phenytoin treatment. The exact mechanism behind this interaction is unknown, but several theories have been explored. One possible explanation is that phenytoin may increase the pH of the small intestine which results in impaired intestinal absorption of folates [55]. Other hypotheses include direct competition between folate and phenytoin for uptake sites, inhibition of folate inter-converting enzymes by phenytoin, and increased catabolism of folates by phenytoin induction of folate catabolic enzymes [55]. There is currently no standard recommendation for the use of folic acid supplementation in patients receiving long term phenytoin therapy, but monitoring of folate levels seems prudent.

Additionally, pharmacological doses of folic acid interact with phenytoin and results in decreased serum concentrations of phenytoin. This interaction is possibly due to direct competition between folate and phenytoin for uptake sites, and be even be severe enough to precipitate seizures [55].

### Vitamin B6 (Pyridoxine)

Vitamin B6, or pyridoxine, is a water-soluble vitamin that has been shown to decrease the effects of phenytoin. Pyridoxine doses of 200 mg/day have been reported to reduce phenytoin concentrations by nearly 50% [56]. The effects of pyridoxine doses lower than 200 mg/day on phenytoin serum concentration have not been established [57].

### Ethanol

Though mild to moderate amounts of ethanol consumption is not expected to affect phenytoin metabolism significantly, acute ethanol ingestion and excess intake inhibits the metabolism of phenytoin and results in increased plasma concentrations of the drug. With chronic alcohol use, ethanol induces hepatic metabolism of phenytoin and results in reduced serum concentrations. Because of this interaction and the fact that ethanol itself may be epileptogenic, chronic consumption increases the risk of seizures and treatment failure.

## FOSPHENYTOIN

Fosphenytoin is a prodrug which is quickly metabolized to pharmacologically active phenytoin after administration. Pharmacokinetics for derived phenytoin are identical to when phenytoin is administered directly. No drugs have been identified that interfere with the conversion of fosphenytoin to phenytoin [23]. Drug–drug interactions for fosphenytoin are the same as those expected to occur with phenytoin [23].

## Conclusion

Of all the antiepileptic medications, phenytoin is associated with the most clinically significant drug interactions. Phenytoin's nonlinear accumulation pattern and unique pharmacokinetics attribute to the high incidence of drug interactions. Phenytoin is highly bound to serum proteins and is a potent inducer as well as a substrate of several drug metabolizing enzymes, making it particularly susceptible to drug interactions due to displacement or metabolic inhibition. Phenytoin undergoes hepatic metabolism mainly by CYP2C9 and slightly by CYP2C19, and drugs that inhibit or induce these enzymes are expected to result in drug interactions. Because only slight changes in metabolism can disproportionately increase phenytoin concentrations, the risk for toxicity is significant. Though the clinical significance of phenytoin drug interactions vary, monitoring of clinical symptoms as well as serum phenytoin concentrations is necessary when a drug interaction is of concern.

## References

[1] Zaccara, G; Perucca, E. "Interactions between Antiepileptic Drugs, and between Antiepileptic Drugs and Other Drugs." *Epileptic Disorders*, 16, no. 4, (December 2014), 409-31.

[2] French, J; Photographer, A; Gidal, BE. "Antiepileptic drug interactions." *Epilepsia,* 41, Suppl 8, (2000), S30-6.

[3] Wilder, Bruce J; Ilo, Leppik; Hietpas, TJ; James, C Cloyd; Edward, J. Randinitis and Judy H Cook. "Effect of food on absorption of Dilantin Kapseals and Mylan extended phenytoin sodium capsules." *Neurology,* 57, 4, (2001), 582-9.

[4] Cacek, AT. "Review of alterations in oral phenytoin bioavailability associated with formulation, antacids, and food." *Therapeutic drug monitoring,* 8, 2, (1986), 166-71.

[5] Haley, CJ; Nelson, J. "Phenytoin-enteral Feeding Interaction." *Annals of Pharmacotherapy*, *23*, no. 10, (October 1989), 796-89.

[6] Patsalos, Philip N; Walter, Froescher; Francesco, Pisani; Clementina, M. van Rijn. "The importance of drug interactions in epilepsy therapy." *Epilepsia,* 43, 4, (2002), 365-85.

[7] Lexicomp Online. *Phenytoin.* 2019. Wolters Kluwer Health, Inc. Accessed June 07, 2019. https://online.lexi.com/.

[8] Nelson, Maureen HS; Angela, K. Birnbaum; Rory, P. Remmel. "Inhibition of phenytoin hydroxylation in human liver microsomes by several selective serotonin re-uptake inhibitors." *Epilepsy Research,* 44, (2001), 71-82.

[9] Brodie, Martin J; Mintzer, SJW; Alison, M. Pack; Gidal, BE; Charles, J. Vecht; Dieter, B Schmidt. "Enzyme induction with antiepileptic drugs: cause for concern?" *Epilepsia,* 54, 1, (2013), 11-27.

[10] Perucca, Emilio. "Clinically relevant drug interactions with antiepileptic drugs." *British journal of clinical pharmacology,* 61, 3, (2006), 246-55.

[11] Finch, Andrew; Peter, Pillans. "P-glycoprotein and Its Role in Drug-drug Interactions." *Australian Prescriber*, 37, no. 4, (2014), 137-39.

[12] Lazarowski, Alberto Jorge; Liliana, A. Czornyj; Fabiana, Lubienieki; Elena Silvia, Girardi; Silvia, Vázquez; Carlos, D'Giano. "ABC transporters during epilepsy and mechanisms underlying multidrug resistance in refractory epilepsy." *Epilepsia,* 48, Suppl 5, (2007), 140-9.

[13] Rivers, Francesca; Terence, J. O'Brien; Richard, Callaghan. "Exploring the possible interaction between anti-epilepsy drugs and multidrug efflux pumps; *in vitro* observations." *European journal of pharmacology,* 598, 1-3, (2008), 1-8.

[14] Löscher, Wolfgang; Dieter, B. Schmidt. "Experimental and clinical evidence for loss of effect (tolerance) during prolonged treatment with antiepileptic drugs." *Epilepsia,* 47, 8, (2006), 1253-84.

[15] Schinkel, Alfred H; Els, Wagenaar; Mol, CA; Liesbeth, Van Deemter. "P-glycoprotein in the blood-brain barrier of mice influences the brain

penetration and pharmacological activity of many drugs." *The Journal of clinical investigation,* 97, 11, (1996), 2517-24.

[16] Potschka, Heidrun; Wolfgang, Löscher. "*In vivo* evidence for P-glycoprotein-mediated transport of phenytoin at the blood-brain barrier of rats." *Epilepsia*, 42, 10, (2001), 1231-40.

[17] Aronica, E; Jan, A. Gorter; Jansen, GH; van Veelen, CWM; Dirk, G. Troost. "Expression and cellular distribution of multidrug transporter proteins in two major causes of medically intractable epilepsy: focal cortical dysplasia and glioneuronal tumors." *Neuroscience,* 118, (2003), 417-429.

[18] Mamiya, Kohsuke; Ichiro, Ieiri; Junta, Shimamoto; Eiji, Yukawa; Jun, Imai; Hideaki, Ninomiya; Hiroaki, Yamada; Kenji, Otsubo; Shun, Higuchi; Nobutada, Tashiro. "The Effects of Genetic Polymorphisms of CYP2C9 and CYP2C 19 on Phenytoin Metabolism in Japanese Adult Patients with Epilepsy: Studies in Stereoselective Hydroxylation and Population Pharmacokinetics." *Epilepsia*, 39, no. 12, (1998), 1317-323.

[19] Caudle, Kelly E; Allan, E Rettie; Michelle, Whirl-Carrillo; Lisa, Noelle; Smith, SJW; Mintzer, Ming Ta Michael Lee; Teri, E. Klein; Thomas Callaghan, J. "Clinical pharmacogenetics implementation consortium guidelines for CYP2C9 and HLA-B genotypes and phenytoin dosing." *Clinical pharmacology and therapeutics,* 96, 5, (2014), 542-8.

[20] Swen, Jesse J; Marga, Nijenhuis; Anthonius, de Boer; Leonora, Grandia; Anke-Hilse, Maitland-van der Zee; Hans, Mulder; Gerard, A. Rongen; Ron, HN. van Schaik; Tom, Schalekamp; Daan, J. Touw; Jan van der, Weide; Bob, Wilffert; Vera, Henriëtte Marie Deneer; Guchelaar, HJ. "Pharmacogenetics: from bench to byte--an update of guidelines." *Clinical pharmacology and therapeutics,* 89, 5, (2011), 662-73.

[21] Delafuente, Jeffrey C. "Pharmacokinetic and pharmacodynamic alterations in the geriatric patient." *The Consultant pharmacist: the journal of the American Society of Consultant Pharmacists,* 23, 4, (2008), 324-34.

[22] Perucca, Emilio; Patrick, Kwan. "Overtreatment in Epilepsy." *CNS Drugs*, 19, no. 11, (2005), 897-908.

[23] Patsalos, Philip N; Edgar, Pathrose Spencer; Dave, Berry. "Therapeutic Drug Monitoring of Antiepileptic Drugs in Epilepsy: A 2018 Update." *Therapeutic drug monitoring,* 40, 5, (2018), 526-548.

[24] Patsalos, Philip N; Emilio, Perucca. Clinically important drug interactions in epilepsy: General features and interactions between antiepileptic drugs. *Lancet Neurology*, 2, (2003), 347-56.

[25] Trojnar, Michał K; Katarzyna, Wojtal; Marcin, Trojnar; Stanisław, Jerzy Czuczwar. "Stiripentol. A novel antiepileptic drug." *Pharmacological reports: PR*, 57, 2, (2005), 154-60.

[26] Perucca, Emilio; James, C Cloyd; David, Critchley; Eliane, Fuseau. "Rufinamide: clinical pharmacokinetics and concentration-response relationships in patients with epilepsy." *Epilepsia,* 49, 7, (2008), 1123-41.

[27] Zhou, Shu-Feng; Charlie, Changli Xue; Xue-qing, Yu; Chunguang, Li; Guangji, Wang. "Clinically important drug interactions potentially involving mechanism-based inhibition of cytochrome P450 3A4 and the role of therapeutic drug monitoring." *Therapeutic drug monitoring,* 29, 6, (2007), 687-710.

[28] Kulshrestha, Vandana; Margaret, Thomas; James, J. Wadsworth; Alan, Richens. "Interaction between phenytoin and antacids." *British journal of clinical pharmacology,* 6, 2, (1978), 177-9.

[29] Carnovale, C; Pozzi, M; Mazhar, F; et al. Interactions Between Antiepileptic and Antibiotic Drugs: A Systematic Review and Meta-Analysis with Dosing Implications. *Clinical Pharmacokinetics,* (2018), 58, 875.

[30] Antoniou, Tony; Tara, Gomes; Muhammad, M Mamdani; David, N Juurlink. "Trimethoprim/sulfamethoxazole-induced phenytoin toxicity in the elderly: a population-based study." *British journal of clinical pharmacology,* 71, 4, (2011), 544-9.

[31] Purkins, Lynn; Nigelo, Wood; Parviz, Ghahramani; Edward, R Love; Malcolm, D. Eve; Anitra, Fielding. "Coadministration of voriconazole

and phenytoin: pharmacokinetic interaction, safety, and toleration." *British journal of clinical pharmacology*, 56, Suppl 1, (2003), 37-44.

[32] Ducharme, Murray P; Richard, L. Slaughter; Lawrence, H. Warbasse; Pranatharthi, Chandrasekar; Veerle Van De, Velde; Geert, SJ Mannens; David, Clive Edwards. "Itraconazole and hydroxyitraconazole serum concentrations are reduced more than tenfold by phenytoin." *Clinical pharmacology and therapeutics,* 58, 6, (1995), 617-24.

[33] Gopal, Krishna; Angela, Sansone-Parsons; Bhavna, S Kantesaria. "Drug interaction assessment following concomitant administration of posaconazole and phenytoin in healthy men." *Current medical research and opinion*, 23, 6, (2007), 1415-22.

[34] Spina, Edoardo; Emilio, Perucca. "Clinical significance of pharmacokinetic interactions between antiepileptic and psychotropic drugs." *Epilepsia,* 43, Suppl 2, (2002), 37-44.

[35] Shin, Jinyoung; Ji-Young, Park; Moon, Young Kim; Shon, JO; Young-Ran, Yoon; In-June, Cha; Sang-Seop, Lee; Se-wook, Oh; Sang-Woo, Kim; David, A. Flockhart. "Inhibitory effects of tricyclic antidepressants (TCAs) on human cytochrome P450 enzymes *in vitro*: mechanism of drug interaction between TCAs and phenytoin." *Drug metabolism and disposition: the biological fate of chemicals*, 30, 10, (2002), 1102-7.

[36] Spaans, E; van den Heuvel, M; Schnabel, P; Peeters, P; Chin-Kon-Sung, U; Colbers, E; Sitsen, J. "Concomitant use of mirtazapine and phenytoin: a drug–drug interaction study in healthy male subjects." *European Journal of Clinical Pharmacology*, 58, (2000), 423-429.

[37] Haselberger, MB; Laurence, S Freedman; Tolbert, SG. "Elevated serum phenytoin concentrations associated with coadministration of sertraline." *Journal of clinical psychopharmacology,* 17, 2, (1997), 107-9.

[38] De Jonge, Milly E; Alwin, DR. Huitema; Selma, M. van Dam; Jos, H. Beijnen; Sjoerd, Rodenhuis. "Significant induction of cyclophosphamide and thiotepa metabolism by phenytoin." *Cancer Chemotherapy and Pharmacology*, 55, (2004), 507-510.

[39] Vecht, Charles J; Louis Wagner, G; Erik, B Wilms. "Interactions between antiepileptic and chemotherapeutic drugs." *The Lancet Neurology*, 2, (2003), 404-409.

[40] Miller, Del D. "Effect of phenytoin on plasma clozapine concentrations in two patients." *The Journal of clinical psychiatry*, 52, 1, (1991), 23-5.

[41] Wong, Yingcong; Chiao, Wen Yeh; Per, Trygve Thyrum. "The effects of concomitant phenytoin administration on the steady-state pharmacokinetics of quetiapine." *Journal of clinical psychopharmacology,* 21, 1, (2001), 89-93.

[42] Nappi, Jean M. "Warfarin and Phenytoin Interaction." *Annals of Internal Medicine*, 90, no. 5, (1979), 852.

[43] Taylor, Jerry W; Bruce, Alexander; Lynn, W. Lyon. "A Comparative Evaluation of Oral Anticoagulant-Phenytoin Interactions." *Drug Intelligence & Clinical Pharmacy*, 14, no. 10, (1980), 669-73.

[44] Galgani, Alessandro; Caterina, Palleria; Luigi, Francesco Iannone; Giovambattista, De Sarro; Filippo, Sean Giorgi; Marta, Maschio; Emilio, Russo. "Pharmacokinetic Interactions of Clinical Interest Between Direct Oral Anticoagulants and Antiepileptic Drugs." *Frontiers in Neurology*, 9, (2018).

[45] Melander, AP; Gunnar, Brante; Johansson, Ö; Tor, Lindberg; Elisabeth, Wahlin-Boll. "Influence of food on the absorption of phenytoin in man." *European Journal of Clinical Pharmacology*, 15, (1979), 269-274.

[46] Boullata, Joseph I; Lauren, M Hudson. "Drug-nutrient interactions: a broad view with implications for practice." *Journal of the Academy of Nutrition and Dietetics,* 112, 4, (2012), 506-17.

[47] Italiano, Domenico; Edoardo, Spina; Jose, de Leon. "Pharmacokinetic and pharmacodynamic interactions between antiepileptics and antidepressants." *Expert opinion on drug metabolism & toxicology*, 10, 11, (2014), 1457-89.

[48] Pennell, Page B. "The importance of monotherapy in pregnancy." *Neurology,* 60, 11, Suppl 4, (2003a), S31-8.

[49] Pennell, Page B. "Antiepileptic drug pharmacokinetics during pregnancy and lactation." *Neurology*, 61, 6, Suppl 2, (2003b), S35-42.

[50] Williams, Nancy Toedter. "Medication administration through enteral feeding tubes." *American journal of health-system pharmacy: AJHP: official journal of the American Society of Health-System Pharmacists*, 65, 24, (2008), 2347-57.

[51] Yeung, SC Au; Mary, HH. Ensom. "Phenytoin and enteral feedings: does evidence support an interaction?" *The Annals of pharmacotherapy,* 34, 7-8, (2000), 896-905.

[52] Beckwith, Michael Bernard; Sarah, S. Feddema; Richard, G. Barton; Caran, P Graves. "A guide to drug therapy in patients with enteral feeding tubes: Dosage form selection and administration methods." *Hospital Pharmacy*, 39, 3, (2004), 225–237.

[53] Gilbert, Steve; Jimmi, Hatton; Barbara, Magnuson. "How to Minimize Interaction Between Phenytoin and Enteral Feedings: Two Approaches." *Nutrition in Clinical Practice*, 11, no. 1, (1996), 28-31.

[54] Phelps, Nicole. "Management of Phenytoin with Enteral Tube Feeding." *Mental Health Clinician*, 2, no. 5, (2012), 108-09.

[55] Nayyar, Abhishek Singh; Byrappa, Nataraju; Subha, GT. "Phenytoin-Folate Interactions: How Far is Safe Folate Supplementation in Phenytoin Treated Epileptic Patients?" *Journal of Applied Pharmaceutical Science*, 2, no 6, (2012), 230-235.

[56] Hansson, O; Sillanpaa, M. "Pyridoxine And Serum Concentration Of Phenytoin And Phenobarbitone." *The Lancet*, 307, no. 7953, (1976), 256.

[57] Ezzo, Danielle; Maria, Marzella Sulli. Drug Interactions with Vitamins and Minerals. *US Pharmacist*, 1, (2007), 42-55.

In: The Pharmacological Guide to Phenytoin ISBN: 978-1-53616-980-5
Editor: Payal Sud 

*Chapter 6*

# TOXICOLOGICAL MANIFESTATIONS

***Vincent Lee**, MD, MA***
Department of Emergency Medicine and Medical Toxicology,
Long Island Jewish Medical Center, North Shore University Hospital,
Manhasset, NY, US

## ABSTRACT

Toxicity from phenytoin overdose is dependent on the route of administration, duration of exposure (acute and chronic), and the dosage. Phenytoin is found in both oral and intravenous formulations and is also available as a water-soluble prodrug, fosphenytoin. Toxicity is manifested when serum levels exceed the therapeutic level, leading to classic cerebellar and vestibular dysfunction with symptoms such as nystagmus, slurred speech, and ataxia. In addition, phenytoin also produces toxicity through the cardiovascular system, gastrointestinal system, skin, gums, hematopoietic system, and liver.

* Corresponding Author's Email: vince.lee.86@gmail.com.

# Oral Phenytoin Toxicity

## Introduction

Oral phenytoin toxicity may occur acutely after ingestions of large intentional or unintentional overdoses. Most patients presenting with unintentional phenytoin intoxication or mild to moderate intentional poisonings exhibit mild toxicity and rarely exhibit serious morbidity or mortality. In contrast, chronic overdoses usually occur iatrogenically in patients with seizure disorders, particularly after medication initiation or adjustments in dosage, but may also be seen with drug interactions, inter-individual variability, genetic mutations in the cytochrome P450 enzymes, or alterations of physiologic state in disease conditions. Since phenytoin concentrates in the tissues of the central nervous system (CNS), toxicity is presented mainly by dysfunctions of the cerebellar and vestibular system [1].

*Acute Oral Phenytoin Overdoses*

Toxicity from acute oral ingestions of phenytoin occurs after exceeding its therapeutic level (10-20 mg/L), with the onset of symptoms generally within hours of overdose. In general, signs of phenytoin toxicity correlate well with serum concentrations and are mainly manifested through cerebellar and vestibular dysfunction. Mild overdoses (15-30 mg/L) present with spontaneous horizontal or vertical nystagmus on lateral gaze, vertigo, and ataxia.

Moderate overdoses (30-50 mg/L) present with worsening nystagmus and ataxia in addition to diplopia, dysarthria, coarse resting tremors, hyperreflexia, and drowsiness. Although rare, movement disorders have been described in case reports and present as hand tremors, clonus, asterixis, dystonia, orofacial dyskinesia, and generalized choreoathetoid movements [2 - 5]. The mechanism is unknown, but may be due to an imbalance between dopaminergic, cholinergic, and serotonergic pathways in the basal ganglia [2 - 5]. Focal neurological signs are also rare, and present as hemiparesis, hemisensory disturbance, and dysphagia [2]. Paradoxical seizures are rare but have been reported in case studies and seem to correlate with phenytoin levels > 30 mg/L [6, 7]. In addition, gastrointestinal symptoms of nausea and vomiting may also occur [4].

Severe overdoses (> 50 mg/L) produce progressively worsening CNS depression such as disorientation, confusion, and lethargy, with rare progression to coma and respiratory depression. It is worthwhile to note that the presence of seizures may be due to the drug itself or from alternative causes such as co-ingestants that may lower the seizure threshold, underlying seizure disorder, chronic disease conditions such as sepsis, metabolic derangements, or withdrawal from drugs or alcohol [1].

Cardiovascular complications, such as arrhythmias and hypotension, and death are unlikely to occur in acute oral overdoses but have been reported in literature [1, 10, 14, 42, 48, 50]. Theoretically, bradyarrhythmias and hypotension may be seen since phenytoin has class IB antiarrhythmic properties, with inhibitory effects on voltage-gated sodium channels in cardiac myocyte and Purkinje fiber cell membranes. This shortens the rate of depolarization of the cardiac action potential and prolongs the refractory period resulting in conduction delays. Arrhythmias reported include bradycardia, ventricular fibrillation, ventricular tachycardia, and asystole [1]. Electrocardiogram complications include increased PR interval, widened QRS interval, and ST-segment and T-wave changes [1]. The cardiac effects of phenytoin may be exacerbated in overdoses, particularly in patients with chronic disease conditions such as cardiomyopathy or sinus node disease [10].

*Srinivasan et al.* describes a 41-year-old woman who developed sinus bradycardia associated with cardiovascular instability after a reported ingestion of 20 grams of oral phenytoin and 500 mg of glyburide [14]. Treatment required high doses of norepinephrine and dopamine infusions and a transvenous pacemaker. A peak phenytoin concentration taken on hospital day 4 was 80 mcg/mL. Of note, hypoglycemia was not seen throughout the patient's hospital course due to a continuous dextrose infusion. The authors attributed the development of cardiotoxicity from glyburide's inhibitory effect on CYP2C9-mediated metabolism of phenytoin and displacement of phenytoin from plasma protein binding sites, leading to its accumulation [1]. A retrospective chart review of 57 patients over 2-years from an inner-city hospital presenting with severe oral phenytoin overdose (defined by peak concentrations > 40 mcg/mL) revealed new electrocardiogram (ECG) abnormalities in 48% of patients [15]. ECG abnormalities include nonspecific ST-T abnormalities, ventricular conduction delay, left-axis deviation, left ventricular hypertrophy, sinus bradycardia, age-indeterminate myocardial infarction, and sinus tachycardia. Mean peak phenytoin levels was 49.4 ± 7.7 mcg/mL and ranged from 40 to 76 mcg/mL. Suicide was mentioned as a motive for seven patients and the overdoses were likely acute in nature. However, none experienced hemodynamic instability or complications requiring medical attention.

Death is a rare complication of oral phenytoin toxicity. According to the American Association of Poison Control Centers' National Poison Data System (NPDS), there were only 2 reported deaths involving oral phenytoin in 2017 [11]. One case involved an acute adverse reaction from oral phenytoin in a 69-year-old female, resulting in a whole blood phenytoin level of 55 mcg/mL taken at an unknown time. The second case was an intentional acute overdose of pentobarbital and phenytoin, with phenytoin contributing to the patient's death. There are only a few case reports describing fatal oral phenytoin overdose. *Laubscher* describes a 4-year-old girl who ingested 40 tablets of 50 mg phenytoin with resultant cardiovascular collapse and cerebellar tonsil herniation 3 days after presentation [8]. Her post-mortem serum phenytoin level of 9.4 mg/100 mL taken 24-hours after presentation. *Tichner et al.* describes a 16-year-old girl who intentionally overdosed on an unknown quantity of phenytoin and presented with coma about 12-hours after reported ingestion. She then progressed to hypotension and atrial fibrillation with rapid ventricular rate complicated with bidirectional ventricular tachycardia after 24-hours. About 41-hours after admission, the patient died and had post-mortem findings of cerebral edema, pulmonary congestion, and severe renal congestion. A phenytoin concentration was not reported. However, the authors contributed the arrhythmias to the combination depressant effect on cardiac conduction by phenytoin and myocardial irritability of the vasopressors (amphetamine, caffeine, and nikethamide) used at the time.

Prolonged phenytoin toxicity and delays in peak serum concentration are expected in large overdoses [16]. During large overdoses, its metabolizing CYP450 enzymes are saturated, and elimination switches to zero-order kinetics, greatly increasing its half-life. [9], altered gastrointestinal absorption, and tendency to form concretions in overdoses. This results in prolonged duration of symptoms and hospitalization with its associated complications [1].

A unique case of acute oral phenytoin toxicity was described by *Roldan et al.* where a 26-year-old male body-stuffer swallowed several rocks of crack cocaine that was unknowingly adulterated with phenytoin in an effort to conceal from police [12]. After about 2 hours, he developed clinical signs of cocaine toxicity and later developed confusion, truncal ataxia, diplopia, slurred speech, and multidirectional nystagmus. A phenytoin level was recommended by poison control after a negative medical workup. His phenytoin level was 48 mcg/mL. Although rare, clinicians should consider the presence of adulterants, including phenytoin, in the differential diagnosis of atypical presentations of cocaine intoxication.

## Acute Toxicity from Inhaled Phenytoin

The first report of phenytoin-adulterated crack cocaine was described by *Katz et al.* in 1993 [13]. They describe 5 cases of phenytoin intoxication. Case 1 was a 40-year-old man with a history of epilepsy and cocaine use who smoked crack cocaine 13 hours prior to presentation that was intentionally adulterated with 60 phenytoin tablets that presented with ataxic gait, slurred speech, tremors, horizontal nystagmus, hyperactive symmetric deep tendon reflexes, dysdiadochokinesis, and abnormal cerebellar testing. Serum phenytoin level was 52 mcg/mL and he was treated with orogastric lavage with multi-dose activated charcoal. The patient's symptoms resolved, and he was discharged about 19 hours later. Cases 2 and 3 were asymptomatic and were acquaintances of patient 1 but had positive serum phenytoin levels of 7 mcg/mL and 8 mcg/mL respectively. Case 4 was a 42-year-old man with history of epilepsy who presented with nystagmus and ataxia 1-hour after smoking crack cocaine mixed with phenytoin. His serum phenytoin level was 22 mcg/mL. Case 5 was a 34-year-old man with history of epilepsy who presented with marked nystagmus, ataxia, and slightly slurred speech shortly after smoking cocaine mixed with phenytoin. His serum phenytoin level was 32 mcg/mL. After leaving against medical advice and presumably smoking additional crack cocaine mixed with phenytoin, the patient returned 6 hours later with nystagmus, ataxia, increased slurred speech, and marked lethargy. His repeat serum phenytoin level was 50 mcg/mL. All patients denied oral ingestion of phenytoin. The motive of adding phenytoin to cocaine was to enhance the effect of intoxication, as the CNS effects of phenytoin were desirable to certain drug abusers. Although the recreational practice of co-abusing cocaine and phenytoin is uncommon, providers should consider phenytoin toxicity in cocaine abusers presenting with lethargy or cerebellar findings.

## Chronic Oral Phenytoin Toxicity

Chronic oral overdoses of phenytoin are frequently seen iatrogenically, occurring unintentionally through dosing adjustments and drug interactions. Circumstances leading to toxicity may be due to errors in prescribing, dispensing, or administration [1, 17-21]. According to the NPDS data in 2017, about 69% of reported single phenytoin exposures were unintentional or due to adverse reactions [11]. The cerebellar-vestibular manifestations of chronic phenytoin toxicity are dose-related, similar to those seen in acute oral overdoses. Additional toxicity may also manifest through the endocrine, integumentary, skeletal, and hematologic systems. Unpredictably, dose-related toxicity may also develop with chronic therapeutic concentration in some patients.

The incidence of cutaneous manifestations in chronic oral phenytoin use ranges from 2 – 19.4% and is non-dose related [22 - 26]. This discrepancy is most likely due to different genetic backgrounds in subsets of population that predispose patients to toxicity [26]. Inflammatory cutaneous adverse effects range from generalized maculopapular eruptions, erythema multiforme, to a generalized exfoliative dermatitis and Stevens-Johnson syndrome/Toxic epidermal necrolysis (SJS/TEN) [31]. Although rare, prolonged phenytoin has been well-associated with developing a variety of collagen vascular-like diseases, including a drug-induced lupus [1]. Common cutaneous non-inflammatory side effects of phenytoin include hirsutism, gingival hyperplasia, and coarse facies [22, 27-29]. Although rare, anticonvulsant hypersensitivity syndrome (AHS), formerly known as drug rash with eosinophilia and systemic symptoms (DRESS) and drug-induced pseudolymphoma, is the most life-threatening cutaneous complication of phenytoin.

Although purple glove syndrome (PGS) is associated with intravenous phenytoin (described in detail later in this chapter), there are cases report describing its development with oral phenytoin [75, 76]. *Yoshikawa et al.* reported a 10-year-old boy (18 kg body weight) with a history of spastic quadriplegia, intellectual disability, and seizure disorder who developed PGS of his bilateral hands and feet. A pharmacy error lead to administration of 1000 mg phenytoin per day instead of the patient's normal prescription of 100 mg per day. Initially, the patient developed drowsiness, nystagmus, and vomiting. Several hours later, the patient developed edema and purple discoloration in his bilateral hands and feet. Four days after the overdose, he became comatose with worsening edema and discoloration of his extremities. His parents discontinued the drug and his swelling and discoloration gradually improved. Upon presentation to the emergency department, the patient was noted to be in renal failure and had a serum phenytoin concentration of 78.12 mcg/mL taken 2 days after drug discontinuation. PGS resolved completely at 11 days. Authors postulate that accumulation of free phenytoin in small veins and capillaries may induce vasoconstriction and micro-thrombus formation in addition to the patient's impaired vascular integrity from his chronic illness [75, 76].

Anticonvulsant hypersensitivity syndrome is a rare yet potentially fatal systemic and idiosyncratic drug-induced reaction and was first described to be associated with phenytoin in 1959 [30]. This syndrome may also occur with the use of other aromatic anti-epileptic medications including carbamazepine, lamotrigine, phenobarbital, primidone. The etiology of AHS is multi-factorial and appear to be due to an autoimmune-like attack produced by the arene oxide metabolites of these anticonvulsants on specific drug-modified proteins of target organs, such as the liver and skin, of susceptible individuals [22, 33]. Patients with AHS have been found to have inadequate detoxification and elimination of these reactive metabolites, resulting in accumulation and toxicity. It may also be associated with reactivation of the human herpesvirus (HHV) 6, HHV-7, cytomegalovirus, and Epstein Barr virus [22, 31]. Risk factors include African American descent, female sex, and having a susceptible first-degree relative [22]. AHS also has an autosomal dominant inheritance pattern [22]. The incidence is estimated to be about 1 in 1000-10,000 exposures and usually occurs within 2 weeks to 2 months after initiation of a triggering drug [22, 31]. The classic presentation includes development of fever, rash, lymphadenopathy, eosinophilia, and systemic involvement. Mortality is high and ranges from 10-20% and is largely due to systemic dysfunction including hepatotoxicity, pneumonitis, myocarditis, pericarditis, nephritis, and colitis [22, 31, 32, 37].

There is marked variability in the presentation of AHS. Fever is the most common manifestation and is found in about 90-100% of exposures [22]. A skin rash is frequently seen in 90% of patients, with the most common presentation as a diffuse maculopapular rash with subsequent desquamation on resolution [22]. However, rashes may also be severe, manifesting as erythroderma, erythema multiforme, and SJS/TEN. Eosinophilia is the most frequently occurring hematologic abnormality and occurs in about 50% of patients [22]. Other hematologic derangements include thrombocytopenia, anemia, agranulocytosis, and atypical lymphocytes with lymphadenopathy that is frequently mistaken for malignant lymphoma [22, 31]. Hepatic dysfunction is the most characteristic organ involved in AHS [34, 35]. This may range from mild transaminitis to fulminant liver failure [22, 31, 34, 35]. Kidney dysfunction is the second most commonly affected organ, presenting as either proteinuria, interstitial nephritis, vasculitis, or acute renal failure [36]. Other reported manifestations include ulcerations in mucosa, carditis, interstitial pneumonitis, pancreatitis, Conjuncitivitis, pharyngitis, splenomegaly, arthralgia, and myalgias [36]. Delayed transient hypothyroidism may occur after several months past the acute presentation [36].

Phenytoin has been associated with the unpleasant development of hirsutism usually within 3 months of initiation of drug therapy. It is characterized as a generalized growth of excessive body hair, occurring mostly on the extensor surfaces of the extremities, trunk, and face. This cosmetic complication is usually reversible and resolves within 1 year upon drug cessation, but occasionally can be persistent [27, 28, 31].

Gingival hyperplasia was initially reported in association with chronic phenytoin use in 1939 [37, 38]. Other anticonvulsants have also been linked and includes valproic acid, carbamazepine, phenobarbital, and vigabatrin. The prevalence ranges from 13-62%, with higher occurrences found in adolescents and children than in adults [39]. It usually appears within the first 3 months of drug-initiation [40]. The mechanism of phenytoin-induced gingival-hyperplasia is multifactorial and includes inflammation from bacterial plaques secondary to poor oral hygiene, increased gingival fibroblasts that are growth sensitive to phenytoin, and phenytoin-induced decrease in folic acid [31, 40]. Phenytoin-induced fibroblasts synthesize a larger amount of total protein and collagen. In addition, polypeptide growth factor (PDGF-B) has been specifically associated with phenytoin-induced gingival hyperplasia [40]. Clinically, severe gingival hyperplasia may be painful and interfere with daily functions such as eating and speaking.

Prolonged use of phenytoin may induce a variety of collagen vascular disorders, particularly lupus-like syndrome [77-82]. In general, phenytoin-induced collagen vascular-like diseases usually occur insidiously in patients who have been taking the drug for years. A diagnosis of phenytoin-induced lupus usually includes the presence of arthralgias, pleural effusion, pericarditis, positive antinuclear antibody (ANA) in a homogenous pattern, antihistone antibodies with complete resolution without recurrence of symptoms after discontinuation of phenytoin [82]. Other collagen vascular disorders associated with phenytoin have been described in case reports and include dermatomyositis [78], systemic anti-neutrophil cytoplasmic antibody positive (ANCA) vasculitis [81], and granulomatous pulmonary vasculitis [80].

Severe cardiotoxicity in chronic phenytoin overdoses are uncommon. A retrospective review of 57 patients that included both severe acute and chronic oral overdoses showed that patients did not develop hemodynamic instability despite concentrations above 40 ug/mL [15]. Another retrospective review of 44 patients with oral phenytoin overdoses (defined as >20 ug/mL) and mean concentrations of 36.7 ± 12.1 ug/mL (range 20-75 ug/mL) showed no clinically significant cardiovascular abnormalities [41].

In contrast, *Thimmisetty et al.* describes a 50-year-old woman with a history of seizure disorder, cerebral palsy, quadriplegia on oral phenytoin 150 mg twice daily for 6 months presenting with a junctional bradycardia and supratherapeutic level of 36.4 ug/mL [42]. Her baseline ECG was noted to be normal sinus rhythm with a normal rate. She became unresponsive with asystole a few hours after admission. Cardiopulmonary resuscitation (CPR) was performed for 2 minutes and return of spontaneous circulation (ROSC) was achieved. The patient became hemodynamically unstable and was subsequently treated with norepinephrine and dopamine infusions and a temporary transvenous pacemaker. After 2 days, the patient was discharged home.

Additionally, *Su et al.* report a 35-year-old man with a history of traumatic intracranial hemorrhage complicated with post-traumatic seizure disorder and vegetative state on 200 mg oral phenytoin twice daily for 5 months who presented with junctional bradycardia and hypotension [43]. His initial serum phenytoin level was 91 mcg/mL and was associated with hypoalbuminemia of 2.3 g/dL, hyponatremia of 121 mEq/L, and hyperkalemia of 5.4 mEq/L. Treatment with dopamine infusion and atropine was ineffective and a temporary transvenous pacemaker was placed. After fluid resuscitation and correction of electrolytes, the patient's ECG improved to a normal sinus rhythm 3 days later. Of note, the patients in the above cases both had chronic disease states which are associated with hypoalbuminemia, further increasing the fraction of free (active) phenytoin and inducing toxicity [44]. The measurement of free-phenytoin levels may be a better correlation to toxicity in chronically ill patients.

Chronic oral phenytoin neurotoxicity has also been described in a 33-year-old woman with a history of seizure disorder after unknowingly using

Chinese proprietary medicines (CPM) containing the anticonvulsants phenytoin, carbamazepine, and valproate confirmed by chromatography [45]. Her home prescriptions included valproate, carbamazepine, and phenobarbital. The patient consumed 3 bottles of the CPM over 1 month for controlling her epilepsy. The CPM were named "Jue Dian Shen Ying Jiao Nang Yi Hao", "Jue Dian Shen Ying Wan", and "Jue Dian Shen Ying Jiao Nang San Hao". She presented with coma but was hemodynamically stable. Serum phenytoin level was 48.5 mg/L, but her carbamazepine, phenobarbital, and valproate levels were not elevated, presumably due to noncompliance. The patient recovered with conservative treatment and was discharged neurologically intact after 10 days. It is notable that metabolism of valproate, carbamazepine, and phenobarbital are reduced in the presence of phenytoin [1]. Furthermore, valproate may have contributed to this patient's presentation since it is known to displace phenytoin from plasma protein binding sites, leading to an increase in free (active) phenytoin [see Chapter 5].

## INTRAVENOUS PHENYTOIN TOXICITY

Intravenous (IV) phenytoin and fosphenytoin overdoses usually occur iatrogenically by excessive administration or rapid infusion in the hospital setting. Fosphenytoin, the water-soluble prodrug of phenytoin, has also been reported to be unintentionally administered in excessive doses secondary to confusion over drug labeling [1, 46]. Neurotoxicity of parenteral phenytoin poisoning follows a dose-related pattern as in oral overdoses, although may be rapid in onset due to higher bioavailability. In comparison to the oral formulation, significant cardiotoxicity is a well-known complication with parenteral administration of phenytoin, fosphenytoin, and the propylene glycol diluent in phenytoin [1, 47-52]. Additionally, extravasation following administration of IV phenytoin or fosphenytoin may produce the rare but serious complication "Purple Glove Syndrome" (PGS) [54-59].

## Acute Intravenous Phenytoin Toxicity

The most notable signs of toxicity from an acute IV phenytoin poisoning are cardiovascular collapse and/or CNS depression. Since the neurotoxicity of phenytoin has been previously described earlier in this chapter, it will not be further discussed. Due to the potential for cardiac arrhythmias and severe hypotension from rapid IV administration, the Food and Drug Administration (FDA) placed a black box warning recommending that rates should not exceed 50 mg/min in adults and 1-3 mg/kg/min (or 50 mg/min, whichever is slower) in pediatric patients. IV phenytoin is prepared by dissolving the drug in a solvent which contains 40% propylene glycol and 10% ethanol and water, with a pH of 11. When treatment with oral phenytoin is not possible, IV phenytoin can be substituted for oral phenytoin at the same total daily dose. Medication errors in miscalculating concentration conversion leading to severe neurotoxicity have been described [53].

The significant cardiovascular complications of acute IV phenytoin administration are well-described and include hypotension, dysrhythmias, ECG abnormalities (prolongation of PR-intervals and QRS-complex, ST-segment and T-wave changes), and cardiopulmonary arrest [60 - 62]. The incidence of cardiac rhythm disturbances ranges from 3.1 - 7.4% [65] in studies examining phenytoin infusion rates from 40 - 50 mg/min [65] against other anticonvulsants. Cardiovascular toxicity appears to be related to a rapid rate of infusion and propylene glycol diluent found in phenytoin preparations. As previously mentioned, phenytoin possesses class IB antiarrhythmic properties, which results in increased myocardial conduction, shortening of the action potential in injured cardiac tissue, and raises the threshold for ventricular fibrillation [50, 60]. In addition, phenytoin's negative inotropic effect can produce hypotension [50]. Excessive propylene glycol has been found to produce cardiotoxicity by enhanced vagal stimulation and directly depressing the myocardium, which result in ECG abnormalities, hypotension, and cardiac dysrhythmias [60, 61]. Thus, the rapid infusion of phenytoin in its diluent results in severe hypotension and ECG abnormalities due to the additive effects of phenytoin and propylene glycol.

A large prospective study examined 200 patients with a history of seizure disorder receiving 500-1500 mg of phenytoin at an infusion rate of 25-50 mg/min in emergency departments [66]. Four dysrhythmic episodes and three bradycardic hypotensive events occurred with no deaths. The rate of all complications almost doubled when infusion rates were > 50 mg/min. The authors suggest administering phenytoin at rates of 40 mg/min or less. Additionally, they recommend a rate of 25 mg/min to be safer for patients with cardiovascular disease and even lower doses for patients older than 50 years. In another large prospective study, phenytoin was administered in doses of 11-25 mg/kg and at a rate of 50 mg/min to 139 patients for treatment of recurrent seizures or prophylaxis for a subarachnoid hemorrhage [67]. Hypotension (although not defined) was the most frequent complication, seen in 24.1% of patients, and required slowing of infusion most frequently in older patients (ranging from 40-80 years old). Respiratory depression only occurred in one patient, a 66-year-old man who required respiratory support for 3 minutes. No patients developed seizures.

A smaller prospective study examining adverse effects of IV phenytoin administer at 15 mg/kg to 42 adults divided into two treatment arms; group 1 (n=26) consisted of patients treated at an infusion rate of 50 mg/min with a mean age of 32 ± 8 years with no history of cardiovascular disease (CAD) and group 2 (n=16) consisted of patients treated at a rate of 25 mg/min with a mean age of 60 ± 9 years with a history of CAD confirmed by previous record and ECG. Despite the lower infusion rates, three patients in group 2 exhibited cardiovascular side effects, with two patients developing hypotension that resolved with treatment discontinuation and one with junctional bradycardia and hypotension that responded to treatment discontinuation and IV fluid bolus. Authors suggest that elderly patients with a history of CAD should receive IV phenytoin at reduced infusion rates.

However, case reports have shown that despite reduced infusion rates of less than 50 mg/min, significant cardiovascular complications may still occur. *York et al.* described two cases of cardiopulmonary arrest following a reduced rate of phenytoin infusion at 35 mg/min [62]. Case 1 was a 68-

year-old man with a history of seizure disorder, pulmonary hypertension, pulmonary fibrosis, biventricular dysfunction with reduced ejection fraction who was treated for seizures with a loading dose of 1 gram of phenytoin sodium given manually at 35 mg/min. About 25 minutes into the infusion, the patient developed bradycardia and hypotension leading to cardiopulmonary arrest. Cardiopulmonary resuscitation and transthoracic pacing were not effective, and the patient died after 30 minutes. Case 2 was a 44-year-old man with history of seizure disorder, ethanol abuse, and cirrhosis of liver, presenting after a seizure. He was treated with 500 mg of phenytoin given at a manual rate of 35 mg/min. About 15 minutes after completion of the infusion, the patient became hypotensive and apneic with a transient second-degree atrioventricular block followed by asystole. Cardiopulmonary resuscitation was unsuccessful, and the patient died after 20 minutes. Post-mortem exam revealed severe hypertrophy and renal congestion with minimal atherosclerotic coronary heart disease. It is worth noting that both patients were given phenytoin at a manual push rate of 35 mg/min, which introduces human administration error. Additionally, the patient in case 1 had co-morbid congestive heart failure which could have made him more vulnerable to cardiovascular complications despite reduced infusion rate. The patient in case 2 had alcoholic cirrhosis and a known hypoalbuminemia state, which would have increased the fraction of free (active) phenytoin resulting in an increased risk of toxicity.

Another case report described by *Citerio et al.* illustrates the significance of genetic polymorphism of CYP2C9, one of the main metabolic pathways of phenytoin [70]. A 41-year-old woman presented with a new onset seizure with findings of a left frontal lobe oligodendroglioma on computed tomography (CT) scan of the brain. Her seizures persisted during her inpatient course, which prompted treatment with 15 mg/kg of IV phenytoin given over 30 minutes. Two hours post-infusion, the patient was apneic and comatose, subsequently developing hypotension and bradycardia. Transthoracic echocardiography was negative for cardiac lesions. Treatment included intubation, multiple dose activated charcoal (MDAC) and hemodynamic support with dopamine and norepinephrine infusions. Her initial phenytoin level was 79 mcg/mL. She recovered fully after 7 days. The patient was found to be heterozygous for the CYP2C9*3 allele, which is known to have an 85% reduction in enzymatic activity and was most likely responsible for her toxic phenytoin levels.

Parenteral fosphenytoin has been deemed a safer alternative to IV phenytoin for treatment of seizures, particularly because its formulation lacks the propylene glycol diluent [1, 71-74]. It is widely considered that fosphenytoin is possesses a safer cardiovascular risk profile than phenytoin. However, several studies have shown that fosphenytoin may cause more cardiovascular effects than previously believed [46, 52, 71-73]. Fosphenytoin can be administered at triple the rate of phenytoin infusion and is associated with less venous irritation and phlebitis [71]. However, *Adams et al.* performed a 5-year retrospective chart review of the Food and Drug Administration's Adverse Event Reporting System databank and revealed 29 reports of adverse cardiac events likely related to fosphenytoin infusion [72]. This included 10 deaths that involved bradycardic dysrhythmias, 5 cases of sinus arrest, 4 cases of atrioventricular block, and 8 cases of asystole. The suggested mechanism of cardiotoxicity includes fosphenytoin's rapid conversion to phenytoin, exerting its pro-dysrhythmic properties. Additionally, unknown metabolites of fosphenytoin may have pro-dysrhythmic properties [71-73]. Fosphenytoin is formulated with a small amount of inorganic phosphate (0.0037 mmol phosphate/mg phenytoin), which may induce transient hypocalcemia resulting in prolonged QT-interval, leading to torsades de pointes, bradycardia, and heart block [46, 52, 71-73].

Both IV phenytoin and fosphenytoin, to a lesser degree, have been associated with the uncommon yet potentially serious complication of purple glove syndrome (PGS) [54-56]. It is characterized by progressive distal limb edema, characteristic purple-blue discoloration, and pain distal to the site of IV administration [1, 54-59]. Although poorly understood, the proposed mechanism involves precipitation of phenytoin due to altered pH or direct vascular injury and vasospasm by infused fluid, with local tissue ischemia leading to extravasation of phenytoin into interstitial tissue [74]. Another mechanism describes the micro-extravasation of highly alkaline phenytoin into the interstitial tissue due to a leakage from a punctured vein or slipped cannula, producing necrosis, vasoconstriction, and micro-thrombosis [56, 74]. Risk factors include comorbid vascular disease, ages > 60 years and < 7 years, and unconscious patients unable to indicate pain at the IV site [59]. It is unclear if higher phenytoin concentrations contribute to a higher risk of PGS.

There are three classic clinical stages of PGS: 1) Initially, there is blue-purple discoloration adjacent to the IV access site, appearing about 2-12 hours post-administration. 2) Fully developed PGS stage occurs about 12-16 hours later and involves worsening edema and discoloration with subsequent blister formation, sloughing, reddish-purple discoloration. 3) Resolution stage of PGS, presenting as a decrease in size of the discolored area and resolved edema [1, 56, 59]. Pain is typically present at all stages, with rare progression to necrosis of the distal extremity, vascular compression, or compartment syndrome [56]. Histopathologic changes include necrosis of the epidermis with sloughing and ulceration, necrosis of the dermis and subcutaneous tissue, thrombotic occlusion of small vessels, edema, and superficial perivascular lymphocytic inflammation [59]. PGS is distinguished clinically from IV extravasation by the presence of purple-blue discoloration and continued progression despite discontinuation of infusion [59]. Recommendations for prevention of PGS include administration through a large bore proximal peripheral IV or central venous access [56].

## Chronic Intravenous Phenytoin Toxicity

Poisonings from prolonged parenteral administration of phenytoin or fosphenytoin is uncommon and presumably would occur in the hospital setting. Toxicity is expected to follow a dose-related pattern as in oral phenytoin overdoses previously described. It is anticipated that neurotoxicity predominates in the chronic setting, as cardiovascular complications typically is related to rapid rates of infusion in the acute setting.

## COMPLICATIONS IN PREGNANCY AND BREASTFEEDING

Fetal hydantoin syndrome is a well-known teratogenic complication of phenytoin use during pregnancy. As such, phenytoin is classified FDA pregnancy category D. Complete classic phenotype occurs in about 5-10% of cases, while about one third manifest as an incomplete syndrome [90]. The treatment of epilepsy with phenytoin during pregnancy is challenging in that the potential teratogenic effects need to be balanced against the maternal and fetal risk associated with uncontrolled seizures [86, 87].

Fortunately, phenytoin is being used less frequently today in women with epilepsy. Characteristic features include distinctive craniofacial abnormalities (hypertelorism, strabismus, ptosis, flat and broad nose bridge, short nose, large and wide mouth, malformed ears, pterygium colli, and microcephaly), developmental delays, underdeveloped nails, and growth deficiencies [83-85]. Congenital heart disease includes pulmonary or aortic vascular stenosis, coarctation of the aorta, patent ductus arteriosus, and ventricular septal defects [90]. It has been shown to be dose-dependent and influenced by factors that either inhibit or enhance phenytoin metabolism. During pregnancy, total concentrations of phenytoin fall by 50-60% with a decline of 20-30% in free (active) phenytoin concentrations due to enhanced metabolism and protein binding [86, 87]. Thus, the mother is at risk of an increased in seizure frequency. Additionally, teratogenicity of phenytoin is mediated by its toxic intermediate oxidative metabolites (epoxides), rather than the parent compound itself. Epoxides are highly reactive and can covalently bond to embryonic or fetal nucleic acids, disrupting normal fetal development. It has been also been seen that women with a greater epoxide hydroxylase activity have a lower fetal incidence of congenital abnormalities [83, 88].

Hemorrhagic disease of the newborn has also been associated with phenytoin use during pregnancy. Proposed mechanism is the induction of fetal microsomal enzymes by phenytoin with a resulting increased in oxidative degradation of vitamin K. Additionally, the amino acid gamma-carboxyglutamic acid is a component of vitamin-K dependent calcium binding protein in bone. This leads to vitamin-K deficiency in the fetus resulting in hemorrhagic and skeletal defects in the newborn [89].

Anticonvulsants are transferred into breastmilk in an inverse relationship to their extent of protein binding. In general, anticonvulsants with low protein binding, low molecular weight, and high lipophilicity are most likely to accumulate in breastmilk [86]. Since phenytoin is more than 90% protein bound and the benefits of breastfeeding outweigh the potential adverse effects of continued phenytoin exposure, women are encouraged to breastfeed due to the low concentrations found in breastmilk [86-88].

## Conclusion

Phenytoin toxicity mainly manifests with neurotoxicity, specifically cerebellar and vestibular dysfunction with CNS depression. Significant cardiovascular instability characterized with hypotension and bradycardia is mainly associated with rapid infusion rates and the propylene glycol diluent in IV phenytoin. Other complications of phenytoin and fosphenytoin use include purple glove syndrome and drug-induced lupus-like disease. Although fosphenytoin is thought to be a safer alternative to IV phenytoin, cardiotoxicity may still be present. Fetal hydantoin syndrome is the main teratogenic complication of phenytoin used during pregnancy.

## References

[1] Craig, S. *Neurocrit Care.* 2005;3: 161. doi: 10.1385/NCC:3:2:161.

[2] Ahmad S, Laidlaw J, Houghton GW, Richens A. Involuntary movements caused by phenytoin intoxication in epileptic patients. *J Neurol Neurosurg Psychiatry.* 1975;38(3):225-31.

[3] McLellan DL, Swash M. Choreo-athetosis and encephalopathy induced by phenytoin. *Br Med J.* 1974;2(5912):204-5.

[4] Shuttleworth E, Wise G, Paulson G. Choreoathetosis and diphenylhydantoin intoxication. *JAMA.* 1974;230(8):1170-1.

[5] Kooiker JC, Sumi SM. Movement disorder as a manifestation of diphenylhydantoin intoxication. *Neurology.* 1974;24(1):68-71.

[6] Chua HC, Venketasubramanian N, Tan CB, Tjia H. Paradoxical seizures in phenytoin toxicity. *Singapore Med J.* 1999;40(4):276-7.

[7] Stilman N, Masdeu JC. Incidence of seizures with phenytoin toxicity. *Neurology.* 1985;35(12):1769-72.

[8] Laubscher FA. Fatal diphenylhydantoin poisoning. A case report. *JAMA.* 1966;198(10):1120-1.

[9] Chua HC, Venketasubramanian N, Tjia H, Chan SP. Elimination of phenytoin in toxic overdose. *Clin Neurol Neurosurg.* 2000;102(1):6-8.

[10] Wang LW, Subbiah RN, Kilborn MJ, Dunn RF. Phenytoin: an old but effective antiarrhythmic agent for the suppression of ventricular tachycardia. *Med J Aust.* 2013;199(3):209-11.

[11] Gummin DD, Mowry JB, Spyker DA, Brooks DE, Osterthaler KM, Banner W8. 2017 Annual Report of the American Association of Poison Control Centers' National Poison Data System (NPDS): 35th Annual Report. *Clin Toxicol (Phila).* 2018;56(12):1213-1415. doi: 10.1080/15563650.2018.1533727.

[12] Roldan CJ. Phenytoin Toxicity from Cocaine Adulteration. *West J Emerg Med.* 2014;15(2):127–130. doi: 10.5811/westjem.2013.12.20010.

[13] Katz AA, Hoffman RS, Silverman RA. Phenytoin toxicity from smoking crack cocaine adulterated with phenytoin. *Ann Emerg Med.* 1993;22(9):1485-7.

[14] Srinivasan G, Wyawahare M, Mathen PG, and Subrahmanyam DK. Life-threatening bradyarrhythmia with oral phenytoin overdose. *J Pharmacol Pharmacother.* 2015; 6(3):179–181. doi: 10.4103/0976-500X.162017.

[15] Wyte CD, Berk WA. Severe oral phenytoin overdose does not cause cardiovascular morbidity. *Ann Emerg Med.* 1991;20(5):508-12.

[16] Albertson TE, Fisher CJ Jr, Shragg TA, Baselt RC. A prolonged severe intoxication after ingestion of phenytoin and phenobarbital. *West J Med.* 1981;135(5):418-22.

[17] Garrettson LK, Jusko WJ. Diphenylhydantoin elimination kinetics in overdosed children. *Clin Pharmacol Ther.* 1974;17:481-491.

[18] Herberg KP. Inadvertent chronic diphenylhydantoin intoxication in a teenage girl. *J South Carolina Med Assoc.* 1972;68:350-353.

[19] Hopkins JJ, Rooney JC. Phenytoin intoxication in childhood due to incorrect prescribing, dispensing and administration of suspensions. *MJA.* 1969;2:278-279.

[20] Bochner F, Hopper JH, Tyrer JH. Factors involved in an outbreak of phenytoin intoxication. *J Neurol Sci.* 1972;16:481-487.

[21] Tyrer JH, Eadie MJ, Sutherlands JM, et al. Outbreak of anticonvulsant intoxication in an Australian city. *BMJ.* 1970;4:271-273.

[22] Ghannam M, Mansour S, Nabulsi A, Abdoh Q. Anticonvulsant hypersensitivity syndrome after phenytoin administration in an adolescent patient: a case report and review of literature. *Clin Mol Allergy.* 2017;15:14. doi: 10.1186/s12948-017-0069-0.

[23] Rapp RP, Norton JA, Young B, Tibbs PA. Cutaneous reactions in head-injured patients receiving phenytoin for seizure prophylaxis. *Neurosurgery.* 1983 Sep;13(3):272-5.

[24] Hebert AA, Ralston JP. Cutaneous reactions to anticonvulsant medications. *J Clin Psychiatry.* 2001;62 Suppl 14:22-6.

[25] Pelekanos J, Camfield P, Camfield C, Gordon K. Allergic rash due to antiepileptic drugs: clinical features and management. *Epilepsia.* 1991;32(4):554-9.

[26] Yang CY, Dao RL, Lee TJ, Lu CW, Yang CH, Hung SI, Chung WH. Severe cutaneous adverse reactions to antiepileptic drugs in Asians. *Neurology.* 2011;77(23):2025-33. doi: 10.1212/WNL.0b013e31823b478c.

[27] Trevisol-Bittencourt PC, da Silva VR, Molinari MA, Troiano AR. Phenytoin as the first option in female epileptic patients?. *Arq Neuropsiquiatr.* 1999;57(3B):784-6.

[28] Livingston S, Petersen D, Boks LL. Hypertrichosis occurring in association with dilantin therapy. *J Pediatr.* 1955;47(3):351-2.

[29] Menon VB, Kurian J, Undela K, Ramesh M, Gowdappa HB. Phenytoin Toxicity: A Case Report. *Journal of Young Pharmacists.* 2015;7(3):272-275. doi:10.5530/jyp.2015.3.20.

[30] Saltzstein S, Ackerman L. Lymphadenopathy induced by anticonvulsant drugs mimicking clinically and pathologically malignant lymphomas. *Cancer.* 1959;12:164-82.

[31] Scheinfeld N. Impact of phenytoin therapy on the skin and skin disease. *Expert Opin Drug Saf.* 2004 Nov;3(6):655-65.

[32] Choudhary S, MD, McLeod M, Torchia D, Romanelli P. Drug Reaction with Eosinophilia and Systemic Symptoms (DRESS) Syndrome. *J Clin Aesthet Dermatol.* 2013; 6(6): 31-37.

[33] Leeder JS. Mechanisms of idiosyncratic hypersensitivity reactions to antiepileptic drugs. *Epilepsia.* 1998;39 Suppl 7:S8-16.

[34] Hiransuthikul A, Rattananupong T, Klaewsongkram J, Rerknimitr P, Pongprutthipan M, Ruxrungtham K5. Drug-induced hypersensitivity syndrome/drug reaction with eosinophilia and systemic symptoms (DIHS/DRESS): 11 years retrospective study in Thailand. *Allergol Int.* 2016;65(4):432-438. doi: 10.1016/j.alit.2016.04.001.

[35] Avancini J, Maragno L, Santi CG, Criado PR. Drug reaction with eosinophilia and systemic symptoms/drug-induced hypersensitivity syndrome: clinical features of 27 patients. *Clin Exp Dermatol.* 2015;40(8):851-9. doi: 10.1111/ced.12682.

[36] Meik S, Arias M, Mego LF, Santoro MCL, Abeldano A, Pallerano G. Anticonvulsant hypersensitivity syndrome (DRESS syndrome): report of 4 cases. *Dermatology Argentina.* 2010;16(4):272-77.

[37] Oelze LL, Pillow MT. Phenytoin-induced drug reaction with eosinophilia and systemic symptoms (DRESS) syndrome: a case report from the emergency department. *J Emerg Med.* 2013 Jan;44(1):75-8. doi: 10.1016/j.jemermed.2011.05.052.

[38] Kimball OP. The treatment of epilepsy with sodium diphenylhydantoinate. *J of the Am Med Assoc.* 1938;112(13):1244-1245.

[39] Majola MP, McFadyen ML, Connolly C, Nair YP, Govender M, Laher MH. Factors influencing phenytoin-induced gingival enlargement. *J Clin Periodontol.* 2000;27(7):506-12.

[40] Corrêa JD, Queiroz-Junior CM, Costa JE, Teixeira AL, Silva TA. Phenytoin-Induced Gingival Overgrowth: A Review of the Molecular, Immune, and Inflammatory Features. *ISRN Dent.* 2011; 2011: 497850. doi: 10.5402/2011/497850.

[41] Evers ML, Izhar A, Aqil A. Cardiac monitoring after phenytoin overdose. *Heart Lung.* 1997;26(4):325-8.

[42] Thimmisetty RK, Gorthi JR, Hazeem MA. Oral Phenytoin Toxicity Causing Sinus Arrest: A Case Report. *Case Rep Cardiol.* 2014;2014:851767. doi: 10.1155/2014/851767.

[43] Su CM, Kung CT, Wang YC, Lu CH. Life-threatening cardiotoxicity due to chronic oral phenytoin overdose. *Neurol India.* 2009;57(2):200-2. doi: 10.4103/0028-3886.51296.

[44] Lindow J, Wijdicks EF. Phenytoin toxicity associated with hypoalbuminemia in critically ill patients. *Chest.* 1994;105(2):602-4.

[45] Lau KK, Lai CK, Chan AW. Phenytoin poisoning after using Chinese proprietary medicines. *Hum Exp Toxicol.* 2000;19(7):385-6.

[46] Presutti M, Pollet L, Stordeur JM, Bruder N, Gouin F. Acute poisoning with phenytoin caused by an error in the administration of fosphenytoin (Prodilantin). *Ann Fr Anesth Reanim* 2000;19: 688-690.

[47] Mathews SR, Badyal DK, Mathew R. Phenytoin-induced bradycardia and hypotension. *Indian J Pharmacol.* 2019; 51(2): 120-122. doi: 10.4103/ijp.IJP_254_17.

[48] Parsai S, Hariri I, Taleb M, Yoon Y. A Literature Review Revisiting Phenytoin-Induced Sinus Arrest. *Am J Ther.* 2016;23(4):e1091-3. doi: 10.1097/MJT.0000000000000159.

[49] Gaies E, Charfi R, Trabelsi S, Salouage I, Lakahl M, Klouz A. Acute phenytoin intoxication: two cases report and literature review. *Therapie.* 2011;66(5):461-3.

[50] Guldiken B, Rémi J, Noachtar S. Cardiovascular adverse effects of phenytoin. *J Neurol.* 2016;263(5):861-870. doi: 10.1007/s00415-015-7967-1.

[51] Lardizabal DV, Lüders HO, Hovinga CA, Bourgeois BF. Severe intoxication after phenytoin infusion: a preventable pharmacogenetic adverse reaction. *Neurology*. 2004;62(1):161.

[52] DeToledo JC, Lowe MR, Rabinstein A, Villaviza N. Cardiac arrest after fast intravenous infusion of phenytoin mistaken for fosphenytoin. *Epilepsia.* 2001;42(2):288.

[53] Lowry JA, Vandover JC, DeGreeff J, Scalzo AJ. Unusual presentation of iatrogenic phenytoin toxicity in a newborn. *J Med Toxicol.* 2005;1(1):26-9.

[54] Hanna DR. Purple glove syndrome: a complication of intravenous phenytoin. *J Neurosci Nurs.* 1992;24(6):340-5.

[55] Garbovsky LA, Drumheller BC, Perrone J. Purple Glove Syndrome after Phenytoin or Fosphenytoin Administration: Review of Reported Cases and Recommendations for Prevention. *J Med Toxicol.* 2015;11(4):445-59. doi: 10.1007/s13181-015-0490-z.

[56] Newman JW, Blunck JR, Fields RK, Croom JE. Fosphenytoin-induced purple glove syndrome: A case report. *Clin Neurol Neurosurg.* 2017;160:50-53. doi: 10.1016/j.clineuro.2017.06.006.

[57] Burneo JG, Anandan JV, Barkley GL. A prospective study of the incidence of the purple glove syndrome. *Epilepsia.* 2001;42(9):1156-9.

[58] Mahajan RP, Batra YK, Rajeev S. Intravenous phenytoin and percutaneous arterial cannulation: the purple-glove syndrome. *Eur J Anaesthesiol.* 2007;24(10):900-1.

[59] Bhattacharjee P, Glusac EJ. Early histopathologic changes in purple glove syndrome. *J Cutan Pathol.* 2004;31(7):513-5.

[60] Hitotsumatsu T, Iwaki T, Fukui M, Tateishi J. Toxic myocardial damage due to intravenous phenytoin administration. *Histopathology.* 1995;26(5):479-80.

[61] Louis S, Kutt H, McDowell F. The cardiocirculatory changes caused by intravenous Dilantin and its solvent. *Am Heart J.* 1967;74(4):523-9.

[62] York RC, Coleridge ST. Cardiopulmonary arrest following intravenous phenytoin loading. *Am J Emerg Med.* 1988;6(3):255-9.

[63] Al-Khudhairi D, Whitwam JG. Autonomic reflexes and the cardiovascular effects of propylene glycol. *Br J Anaesth.* 1986; 58(8):897-902.

[64] Donovan PJ, Cline D. Phenytoin administration by constant intravenous infusion: selective rates of administration. *Ann Emerg Med.* 1991; 20(2):139-42.

[65] Siebert WJ, McGavigan AD. Requirement for cardiac telemetry during intravenous phenytoin infusion: guideline fact or guideline fiction?. *Intern Med J.* 2013; 43(1):7-17. doi: 10.1111/j.1445-5994. 2012.02935.x.

[66] Earnest MP, Marx JA, Drury LR. Complications of intravenous phenytoin for acute treatment of seizures. Recommendations for usage. *JAMA.* 1983; 249(6):762-5.

[67] Cranford RE, Leppik IE, Patrick B, Anderson CB, Kostick B. Intravenous phenytoin: clinical and pharmacokinetic aspects. *Neurology.* 1978; 28(9 Pt 1):874-80.

[68] Beenen LF, Lindeboom J, Kasteleijn-Nolst Trenité DG, Heimans JJ, Snoek FJ, Touw DJ, Adèr HJ, van Alphen HA. Comparative double blind clinical trial of phenytoin and sodium valproate as anticonvulsant prophylaxis after craniotomy: efficacy, tolerability, and cognitive effects. *J Neurol Neurosurg Psychiatry.* 1999; 67(4): 474-80.

[69] Treiman DM, Meyers PD, Walton NY, Collins JF, Colling C, Rowan AJ, Handforth A, Faught E, Calabrese VP, Uthman BM, Ramsay RE, Mamdani MB. A comparison of four treatments for generalized convulsive status epilepticus. Veterans Affairs Status Epilepticus Cooperative Study Group. *N Engl J Med.* 1998; 339(12):792-8.

[70] Citerio G, Nobili A, Airoldi L, Pastorelli R, Patruno A. Severe intoxication after phenytoin infusion: a preventable pharmacogenetic adverse reaction. *Neurology.* 2003; 60(8):1395-6.

[71] Kim HK, Hwang IG, Koh IS, Kim DW. Incidence and risk factors of hypotension after intravenous fosphenytoin administration. *J Clin Pharm Ther.* 2017; 42(5):561-566. doi: 10.1111/jcpt.12537.

[72] Adams BD, Buckley NH, Kim JY, Tipps LB. Fosphenytoin may cause hemodynamically unstable bradydysrhythmias. *J Emerg Med.* 2006; 30(1):75-9.

[73] Boucher BA, Feler CA, Dean JC, Michie DD, Tipton BK, Smith KR Jr, Kramer RE, Young B, Parks BR Jr, Kugler AR. The safety, tolerability, and pharmacokinetics of fosphenytoin after intramuscular and intravenous administration in neurosurgery patients. *Pharmacotherapy.* 1996; 16(4):638-45.

[74] Sharief N, Goonasekera C. Soft tissue injury associated with intravenous phenytoin in a neonate. *Acta Paediatr.* 1994; 83(11): 1218-9.

[75] Yoshikawa H, Abe T, Oda Y. Purple glove syndrome caused by oral administration of phenytoin. *J Child Neurol.* 2000;15(11):762.

[76] Jain RS, Nagpal K, Kumar S, Prakash S, Handa R5. Purple glove syndrome occurring after oral administration of phenytoin in therapeutic doses: mechanism still a dilemma. *Am J Emerg Med.* 2015; 33(1):123.e5-6. doi: 10.1016/j.ajem.2014.05.039.

[77] Ross S, Ormerod AD, Roberts C, Dwyer C, Herriot R. Subacute cutaneous lupus erythematosus associated with phenytoin. *Clin Exp Dermatol.* 2002; 27(6):474-6.

[78] Dimachkie MM, Vriesendorp FJ, Heck KA. Phenytoin-induced dermatomyositis: case report and literature review. *J Child Neurol.* 1998; 13(11):577-80.

[79] Atwater BD, Ai Z, Wolff MR. Fulminant myopericarditis from phenytoin-induced systemic lupus erythematosus. *WMJ.* 2008; 107(6):298-300.

[80] Kheir F, Daroca P, Lasky J. Phenytoin-Associated Granulomatous Pulmonary Vasculitis. *Am J Ther.* 2016; 23(1):e311-4. doi: 10.1097/ MJT.0000000000000006.

[81] Parry RG, Gordon P, Mason JC, Marley NJ. Phenytoin-associated vasculitis and ANCA positivity: a case report. *Nephrol Dial Transplant.* 1996; 11(2):357-9.

[82] Siragusa RJ, Ramos-Caro FA, Edwards NL, Flowers FP. Drug-Induced Lupus Due to Phenytoin. *Journal of Pharmacy Technology.* 2000; 16(1):5-7. doi: 10.1177/875512250001600103.

[83] Buehler BA, Delimont D, van Waes M, Finnell RH. Prenatal prediction of risk of the fetal hydantoin syndrome. *N Engl J Med.* 1990; 322(22):1567-72.

[84] Finnell RH, Buehler BA, Kerr BM, Ager PL, Levy RH. Clinical and experimental studies linking oxidative metabolism to phenytoin-induced teratogenesis. *Neurology.* 1992; 42(4 Suppl 5):25-31.

[85] Loughnan PM, Gold H, Vance JC. Phenytoin teratogenicity in man. *Lancet.* 1973; 1(7794):70-2.

[86] Sabers A, Tomson T. Managing antiepileptic drugs during pregnancy and lactation. *Current Opinion in Neurology.* 2009;22(2):157-161. doi: 10.1097/WCO.0b013e32832923d7.

[87] Pennel PB. Antiepileptic drug pharmacokinetics during pregnancy and lactation. *Neurology.* 2003; 61(Suppl 2):35-42.

[88] Hill DS, Wlodarczyk BJ, Palacios AM, Finnell RH. Teratogenic effects of antiepileptic drugs. *Expert Rev Neurother.* 2010; 10(6): 943-959. doi:10.1586/ern.10.57.

[89] Keith DA, Gallop PM. Phenytoin, hemorrhage, skeletal defects and vitamin K in the newborn. *Med Hypotheses.* 1979; 5(12):1347-51.

[90] Hegde A, Kaur A, Sood A, Dhanorkar M, Varma HT, Singh G, Saini AG, Kumar P. *Fetal Hydantoin Syndrome. J Pediatr.* 2017;188:304. doi: 10.1016/j.jpeds.2017.05.018.

In: The Pharmacological Guide to Phenytoin ISBN: 978-1-53616-980-5
Editor: Payal Sud 

*Chapter 7*

# DIAGNOSIS AND TREATMENT OF TOXICITY

***Tatiana Carrillo[1], DO, Javier Sanchez[1], DO and Angela Regina[2,*], DO***

[1]Department of Emergency Medicine, St. Barnabas Health System, Bronx, NY, US

Department of Emergency Medicine and Medical Toxicology, St. Barnabas Health System. Bronx, NY, US

## ABSTRACT

Phenytoin is a widely used antiepileptic medications and considered the first line treatment in most seizure disorders. With its popular use in the population, the ability to detect and manage its toxicity are important skills for all physicians. Although concentrations of the drug are available through laboratory analysis, the physician must have a high index of suspicion first, as the physician needs to know when to send the sample for analysis. Certain physical exam findings can assist in determining if toxicity is present. In addition to overdose, the Purple Glove Syndrome is one specific adverse effect of phenytoin that must be considered and discussed, which has decreased in incidence since the development of a more water-soluble prodrug fosphenytoin. Once the diagnosis of toxicity

* Corresponding Author's Email: areginatox@gmail.com.

is established, the treatment remains largely supportive, with hemodynamic, respiratory, mental status and neurologic monitoring. Deaths are rare, even after massive overdoses. Multi dose activated charcoal (MDAC) can enhance clearance of the drug from the body, with questionable effect on the clinical manifestations. There is a limited role for extracorporeal treatments in phenytoin toxicity, with specific recommendations and guidelines established. Disposition depends on the clinical scenario, with frequent neurological assessments required in those displaying neurotoxicity. Cardiotoxicity typically only occurs with intravenous (IV) phenytoin and requires cardiac monitoring, but this rarely occurs after an oral overdose. [1]

## INTRODUCTION

The following chapter will discuss the diagnosis and treatment of phenytoin and fosphenytoin toxicity. Specific physical exam findings can give clues that an overdose has occurred and toxicity is present. Laboratory analysis to determine the concentration of the drug in serum can be sent, and used in context with the physical exam findings and the patient's overall clinical condition. Management of toxicity is largely supportive, although MDAC can be considered in certain situations. The extracorporeal treatment in poisoning workgroup (EXTRIP) workgroup has made recommendations for the use of hemodialysis (HD) in phenytoin poisonings. Disposition of the patient must be taken in clinical context, with cardiac monitoring typically only needed with intravenous overdoses and rarely required in oral overdoses.

## DIAGNOSIS OF PHENYTOIN TOXICITY

With most cases of intentional and unintentional overdoses, the patient's history is the most important clue to determining what has occurred. Important historical information that should be obtained is the drug or drugs ingested, the formulation of the drug, including sustained or immediate release preparations, the time of ingestion and amount ingested. A patient may be forthcoming with the pharmaceutical product they have taken, or there may be family, friends or other collaterals who can provide that information. Clinicians, ancillary staff and clinical pharmacists involved in the case can also assist by querying the patient's medical record or their local pharmacy for their medication list. However, there are situations where a history is impossible to obtain, due to either lack of knowledge by the patient, inability to communicate due to altered mental status or the patient refusing to give the information. When the medication and amount ingested are unknown, diagnosis may be more challenging but not impossible. In a situation where a complete medication list is unavailable, the clinician must depend on their skills as a diagnostician. Vital sign interpretation and a thorough physical exam are important and essential tools in determining toxicity from any drug.

Phenytoin is primarily a neurotoxin, without significant effects on hemodynamics. Vital signs are not expected to be deranged during an oral overdose, and should be expected to be within the normal range. [1] Hypotension can be seen with rapid administration of the intravenous solution and is due to the sodium channel-blocking effects of the drug. It impairs myocardial contractility, decreases peripheral vascular resistance and depresses cardiac conduction. Patients who are to be administered IV phenytoin should be placed on a cardiac monitor with frequent blood pressure analysis performed.

With only a couplc of casc rcports documcntcd, bradycardia and hypotension have been rarely seen with phenytoin oral overdoses. The first case of a patient developing bradycardia and hypotension believed to be attributed to phenytoin was in 2005. A 35-year-old male with a history of traumatic intracranial hemorrhage and in a vegetative state was brought to the emergency department (ED) with bradycardia of 35 beats per minute and hypotension of 87/75 mm Hg. He had been on phenytoin for the last 5 months and was also on anti-tuberculous (anti-TB) medications for the last four months. His medications were administered to him, and there was no indication of overdose or misuse of the medications to cause his symptoms. The patient had a transvenous pacemaker implanted and was started on a dopamine infusion. His anti-TB medications were discontinued, he improved and was discharged on day 14 at a return to his baseline. The second report in 2015 was of a 41-year-old female who ingested 20 g of phenytoin along with 500 mg of glibenclamide, a second-generation sulfonylurea used in the management of diabetes mellitus. She developed sinus bradycardia and significant hypotension, requiring noradrenaline and dopamine infusions. She was also intravenously paced. Her hospital course improved, with extubation on day 6 and discharge on day 12 without any neurologic sequelae. [3] In both of these cases of hemodynamic instability related to phenytoin, a second agent could have been a confounding factor. Given the paucity of reports of documented hemodynamic compromise with oral phenytoin overdoses and confounders in the published reports of these cases, hemodynamic monitoring is generally not recommended in oral phenytoin overdoses. [1]

As a neurotoxin, phenytoin affects the cerebellar and vestibular systems resulting in specific physical exam findings, which are established and documented. The cerebellum coordinates unconscious regulation of balance, muscle tone and coordination of voluntary movements. An insult to the cerebellar system would be expected to produce specific findings on the physical exam. These include nystagmus, inability to perform a finger to nose test, inability to perform rapid alternating movements. Gait is often affected as well, and described as a wide base and staggering gait. A neurologic exam should be performed on all patients, but when suspecting phenytoin toxicity it is even more prudent to be complete and thorough. Their mental status, level of consciousness and orientation with their surroundings should be noted. Extraocular muscles should be assessed and any nystagmus documented. Importantly coordination, ability to perform fast alternating hand movements and gait should be tested. Abnormalities to these aspects of the physical exam would provide a high suspicion to toxicity from phenytoin. [4]

Once toxicity from phenytoin is suspected, either from the history or physical exam, a concentration of the drug can be obtained from blood samples from the patient. Given the known pharmacokinetics of phenytoin, signs of acute toxicity can present at various serum concentration levels [see Chapter 4]. Therapeutic concentrations are 10 to 20 mg/L. Traditionally, levels of 15 mg/L and greater are associated with nystagmus, levels above 30mg/L with ataxia and poor coordination, and at levels greater than 50mg/L toxicity may present as slurred speech and extrapyramidal symptoms among other physical findings. [5] Although these numbers are helpful to guide clinicians, it must be noted that patients with impaired or decreased protein binding capacity will manifest toxicity while within the therapeutic range, which will be discussed below. Because of its unpredictable absorption, concentrations should be repeatedly monitored. Concentrations should be drawn every 4 to 6 hours. Trends should be established, both rising and falling, and coordinated with the physical exam during monitoring and treatment. Due to phenytoin's zero order elimination kinetics during an overdose, high serum phenytoin concentrations may take days to weeks to return to therapeutic range. [5]

Phenytoin has a high affinity to serum proteins, mostly albumin and its high protein binding plays an integral component in the manifestation of toxicity. This is especially important in patients that are in hypoalbuminemic states, as often seen in those who are critically ill [see Chapter 3]. As mentioned above, a patient with low protein binding capability can manifest toxicity while still within the therapeutic range, as the serum concentration being measured is the total phenytoin concentration, however the pharmacologically active component is the free phenytoin. In hypoalbuminemic states, the bound fraction will be decreased, while the unbound, and hence active, fraction will be increased, despite a potentially normal total concentration. [5]

Therapeutic free phenytoin concentrations are 1 to 2 mg/L. Patients at greatest risk of toxicity include neonates, elderly adults, hypoalbuminemic, hyperbilirubinemic and uremic patients; and those undergoing combination therapy with valproic acid, salicylates and sulfonamides because these medications displace phenytoin from its albumin binding sites [see Chapter 3]. [5] A series of case reports done by Lindow et al. appreciated acute phenytoin toxicity in ICU patients who received doses of phenytoin between 300 mg and 1500 mg, with free phenytoin levels ranging from 4.4 mg/L - 6.3 mg/L. In all four case reports done by this group the patients were found to have a profound decrease in their albumin levels. It was then observed that with critically ill patients, and those with decreased albumin, the free phenytoin levels were more accurate in assessing toxicity versus total levels. They also determined that serum albumin levels are an integral piece in dosing phenytoin in the critically ill patient with a seizure disorder. The toxic manifestations were consistent with other populations, including cerebellar symptoms, diplopia, nystagmus and emesis. [6]

A correction formula, The Sheiner-Tozer Equation can be utilized in this specific patient population, which approximates the total phenytoin concentration that would be expected on a given measured serum phenytoin concentration and measured albumin concentration:

$$[\text{Phenytoin}] = \frac{[\text{Measured phenytoin}]}{(0.25 \times [\text{Measured albumin}]) + 0.1}$$

This formula should be used for any patient with a low measured albumin (<3.2 g/dL) where typical therapeutic phenytoin ranges are less accurate in determining toxicity. The equation utilizes an adjustment of 0.275 for those patients with a creatinine clearance less than 20 mL/min.

Additionally, other medications such as antibiotics and antifungal will compete with phenytoin for active binding sites, making the usual doses of phenytoin potentially toxic [see Chapter 4]. It is important to consider drug-drug interaction when prescribing additional medications to patients on phenytoin, as there is the potential to alter the kinetics of the drug, leading to toxicity. Cadle et al. reported two cases of fluconazole induced phenytoin toxicity. Fluconazole inhibits CYP-450 and has a predisposition to lead to hepatotoxicity. This requires vigilant monitoring of free phenytoin levels, even at low doses of fluconazole, and recommendations are given for phenytoin monitoring even at doses of 200 mg. [6] Ciprofloxacin is another medication that can potentially alter phenytoin kinetics and concentrations. Pollack et al. discussed a case of a 61-year-old male with a history of seizures on phenytoin 100mg three times a day and recently started on ciprofloxacin for community acquired pneumonia. The patient was found to have serum phenytoin levels of 2.5 mg/L after ciprofloxacin initiation.

Given decrease in serum phenytoin, the dose was titrated up while being treated and the patient was discharged on 200 mg three times a day. The patient went on to develop severe ataxia with serum phenytoin levels of 42 mg/L. Co-administration of ciprofloxacin while on phenytoin was thought to decrease serum concentrations of phenytoin. Although not fully clear, the authors believed this was due to either inhibition of the absorption of phenytoin, or the induction of its metabolism. [7] There are also concerns for drug interactions which can decrease the clearance of phenytoin, leading to toxicity. TMP/SMX co-administration with phenytoin, especially in the elderly has been shown to reduce hepatic metabolism of phenytoin, via the potent inhibition of CYP2C8 by TMP/SMX, causing an almost 30% decrease in clearance of phenytoin during co-administration. [8] This can lead to a chronic toxicity due to decreased clearance of the drug, and close monitoring for adverse effects is recommended.

Although phenytoin has predictable clinical manifestations with toxicity, it is not uncommon for atypical presentations to manifest, especially in elderly patients and children. This is due to their ability to metabolize and clear the drug, leading to various physical exam findings [see Chapter 3]. Marin et al. documented visual hallucinations and constellation of symptoms mimicking delirium tremens in a 4-year-old child with a history of febrile seizures and complex partial seizures. In this case the patient was started on a loading dose of 15mg/kg of phenytoin followed by a maintenance dose of 5mg/kg/day. The visual hallucinations were reported 2 hours after the first dose of phenytoin was administered. The patient reported visualizing small insects with associated tactile abnormalities. Initial phenytoin levels were noted to be subtherapeutic at 6.6 mg/L, but symptoms resolved once phenytoin was discontinued. [9] Shores et al. also documented similar findings in a 71-year-old male. The patient was admitted to the neurology service after experiencing a seizure. He admitted to drinking 2 or 3 beers daily, with his last drink 4 days prior. He was started on 300 mg phenytoin and began to complain of visual hallucinations shortly after the first dose. He described the hallucinations as objects changing in size, and the appearance of the objects vibrating. An EEG was performed and was without abnormalities. A phenytoin level was drawn after the second dose and measured at 5.4 mg/L. The phenytoin was changed to carbamazepine and visual symptoms resolved the next day. [10]

As previously discussed, there are certain populations at a higher risk for toxicity. This increased risk also extends to those patients who use illicit and mind altering substances. Users of cocaine have been noted to present with acute phenytoin toxicity after insufflating crack-cocaine. Katz et al. presented five case reports of individuals presenting to the ED with altered mental status, ataxia, and nystagmus. In each case, phenytoin levels were measurable in the toxic range at 48 mg/L. [11] The cause for this interaction is unknown. Heavy alcohol consumption has also been noted to be a predisposing factor in developing acute phenytoin toxicity. Polman et al. presented a case report of a middle-aged male with history of chronic alcohol use (reported about 6 units daily) admitted for seizures secondary to trauma. The patient was given a phenytoin loading dose of 1000 mg IV followed by maintenance dose of 150 mg twice a day. The patient was reported to develop renal failure and diffuse bilateral pulmonary infiltrates, and it was noted that the initial chest x-ray performed prior to phenytoin administration was without abnormalities. The patient was then believed to be in renopulmonary syndrome, due to the decline in kidney function and pulmonary findings. This was initially thought to be due to Wegener's granulomatosis or Good-pasture's syndrome but these conditions were excluded during his admission. Phenytoin was discontinued on day 9, and symptoms normalized by day 18, and the clinical team determined that his renopulmonary syndrome was due to the phenytoin. [12]

Additionally, cases of phenytoin toxicity have been reported with the use of the drug for seizure prophylaxis in patients with intracranial masses and traumatic injuries. There are uncommon cases of this toxicity mimicking severe acute psychosis and cerebellar syndrome. Agrawal et al. discussed acute psychosis in a phenytoin naïve patient who presented with horizontal nystagmus, acute agitation/aggression, and delusions 10 days after initiating a regimen of 300 mg of phenytoin. [13] Phenytoin was initiated after a diagnosis of Glioblastoma Multiforme. In this specific case phenytoin levels were noted to be >40 mg/L. Symptoms resolved was phenytoin was discontinued.

Furthermore, prolonged oral intake of phenytoin has been shown to present with cutaneous manifestations; cases ranging from maculopapular rash to Drug Rash with Eosinophilia and Systemic Symptoms (DRESS syndrome). Stevens-Johnson Syndrome (SJS) and Toxic epidermal necrolysis (TEN) have been reported as well. [14] There appears to be a genetic component to the development of these cutaneous manifestations, specifically with CYP2C variants. These CYP variants are believed to alter and reduce phenytoin clearance and place the patient at higher risk of severe cutaneous adverse effects described above.

For patients within the hospital setting, an adverse effect that can occur with intravenous phenytoin that must be known about is the Purple glove syndrome (PGS). PSG is a rare complication associated with the use of intravenous phenytoin and fosphenytoin. It typically presents with pain, edema and discoloration at the injection site that then spreads to the distal limb. Risk factors associated with the development of purple glove syndrome are advanced age with pre-existing vascular disease and the use of small gauge catheters for infusion. Fosphenytoin is the water-soluble prodrug of phenytoin, which is considered less toxic than phenytoin, especially if extravasation were to occur. Fosphenytoin has basically replaced intravenous phenytoin due to its favorable toxic profile via this route of administration. Inadvertent overdoses of fosphenytoin are expected to produce a similar clinical picture to phenytoin. As fosphenytoin is not available for outpatient use, intentional overdoses of fosphenytoin are rarer than those of phenytoin.

When initially assessing patients for possible phenytoin toxicity, total serum phenytoin levels, free serum phenytoin levels, serum albumin levels, and electrolytes specifically calcium should be analyzed. Unfortunately, free serum phenytoin levels are not routinely available in most hospital laboratories. Phenytoin directly decreases calcium absorption, leading to hypocalcemia. In cases of de novo seizures from phenytoin itself, other causes of new onset seizures should be excluded first, including metabolic derangements, new ischemic stroke, acute alcohol withdrawal among others, as seizures from phenytoin toxicity are rare. [15]

## TREATMENT OF PHENYTOIN TOXICITY

Once a patient is determined to have toxicity from phenytoin, whether it is from an acute or chronic overdose, therapeutic misadventure, medication interaction or any other etiology, the next step is the management and disposition of the patient. Currently, there is no antidote for phenytoin, and patients presenting to the ED require mainly supportive care, with hemodynamic, respiratory and mental status monitoring. [17] Although oral phenytoin overdoses are not expected to cause cardiovascular compromise as discussed, there should always be a index of suspicion for co-ingestants. If the patient remains hemodynamically stable during the ED assessment and workup, continued telemetry and hemodynamic monitoring will not be required if the patient is felt to require admission to the hospital. As with all cases of intentional or unintentional ingestions and toxicity from medications, attention should initially be focused on initial stabilization. Airway, breathing and circulation, the ABCs, should be assessed and derangements corrected. An advanced airway may be required if the patient cannot protect their airway or if breathing is compromised. Circulation should be assessed and vital signs interpreted. In addition to stabilizing the patient, fall precautions should be instituted, as the potential for traumatic injuries is high considering the loss of coordination that develops.

Cardiotoxicity is rare and typically only occurs through the IV route as discussed above, with only two cases reports of hemodynamic compromised after oral ingestion. Signs of cardiotoxicity include hypotension, EKG changes such as shortened PR interval or prolonged QT interval and cardiac bradydysrrthymias. Cardiotoxicity is normally transient and resolves on its own with cessation of the infusion and fluid administration. [17] Intravenous infusion rates greater than 50mg/min were associated with increased adverse effects. [18] Stopping the phenytoin infusion for a few minutes and administering fluid boluses of 250 to 500 ml of 0.9% sodium chloride solution is generally sufficient to treat hypotension. If infusion is still required after resolution, it is recommended to restart at half of the initial dose. Oral administration of phenytoin does not typically result in any cardiovascular complications, except in rare case reports, so patients who overdose on oral phenytoin typically do not require cardiac monitoring in the ED or during hospitalization. [1, 19]

Those patients presenting with cutaneous manifestations of phenytoin toxicity, especially those with life threatening syndromes such as SJS, should immediately have their medication discontinued, as the mainstay of treatment involves stopping the medication. Consultation with a burn specialist is a consideration with more severe cases of DRESS, SJS and TENS.

If a patient who has acutely overdosed on phenytoin presents to the ED within an hour of presentation, activated charcoal (AC) could be administered to bind to phenytoin, decreasing its systemic absorption. [20] The mental status of the patient and potential coingestants should be taken into account if this treatment modality is utilized. Only those willing and able to drink the activated charcoal should be considered, as patients with a depressed mental status are at a risk for aspiration, and aspiration of charcoal can lead to a severe chemical pneumonitis. This is a significant concern as the chemical pneumonitis can lead to adult respiratory distress syndrome (ARDS) with significant morbidity and mortality. As phenytoin overdose is rarely fatal, aspiration of charcoal would be considered potentially more serious than the initial overdose.

Multi-dose activated charcoal (MDAC) is a technique used to enhance the elimination of certain amenable drugs. The use of charcoal in this treatment modality is not to decrease absorption, but rather to enhance the elimination of the drug via enterohepatic recirculation. This concept of GI or gut dialysis is based on the theory that MDAC enhances the diffusion of the drug from the blood into the GI tract and traps it there for later fecal excretion. In this manner, AC is said to perform as an “infinite sink”, allowing for “gastrointestinal dialysis” to occur. Although MDAC is controversial in the treatment of phenytoin toxicity, it has been shown to reduce the half-life of IV phenytoin in half. [15] MDAC was also shown to reduce serum phenytoin levels more rapidly in those treated with MDAC than in those who weren’t treated with MDAC in patients with supratherapeutic phenytoin levels. [21] In one study, 17 patients were enrolled, all with supratherapeutic levels of phenytoin. Seven of them received MDAC and eight of them served as controls. In this study, the time to reach a therapeutic level was found to be halved in those who received MDAC compared to those who did not. [21] However, it must be mentioned that a decreased serum level does not always correlate to an improvement in clinical condition or ultimate outcomes. In the above mentioned study of 15 adult patients with supratherapeutic phenytoin concentrations, MDAC reduced the time to phenytoin concentration less than 25 mg/L from 41.1 to 19.3 hours, although clinical endpoints were unchanged. Always keep in mind the risk of aspiration in those with a depressed mental state when administering activated charcoal, both in a single dose or through the use of MDAC. In these patients, it is better to secure the airway prior to its administration, although a patient should not be intubated solely for the administration of AC or MDAC. Dosing for MDAC varies, but commonly 50g is given initially followed by 25g every 2 to 4 hours. The optimal single-dose activated charcoal (SDAC) and MDAC dose is unknown. However, it is recommend to administer a minimum AC dose of 1 g/kg of body weight or a 10:1 ratio of AC to drug, up to an amount that can be tolerated by the patient and safely administered if the dose is known, which usually represents 50 to 100 g in adults. AC often comes premixed, but if that is not available, it is best administered as a slurry in a 1:8 ratio of AC to suitable liquid, such as water or cola. Sorbitol containing solutions should be avoided with multiple doses of charcoal, as they can lead to diarrhea and subsequent electrolyte disturbances. The initial dose of activated charcoal can contain sorbitol, but repeated administration of this additive should be avoided for reasons stated above.

Another treatment for phenytoin toxicity is the use of extracorporeal techniques for the removal of the drug. There is conflicting data on the efficacy of hemodialysis and other forms of extracorporeal procedures for elimination, with some case reports showing improved patient outcomes while others showing no change in clinical outcomes. The extracorporeal treatment in poisoning workgroup (EXTRIP) is a group of researchers from many different fields of medicine, including nephrology, medical toxicology, emergency medicine, pharmacology and others who work to systematically review the literature on extracorporeal treatments (ECTR) in poisoned patients. The literature is not limited by date or language, as they have multiple translators on staff. Based on the data reviewed, they have made recommendations on the use of extracorporeal methods of treatment in poisoned patients. Their general recommendation for ECTR is that it would be reasonable in selected cases of severe phenytoin poisoning. Intermittent HD is the preferred method of ECTR, and intermittent hemoperfusion is an acceptable alternative. The indications for HD include prolonged coma present or expected and prolonged incapacitating ataxia that is present or expected. HD is not recommended solely based on the suspected dose of phenytoin ingested or solely on the total serum phenytoin concentration resulted. [22]

One case report showed significant reduction of phenytoin levels by using Molecular Adsorbents Recirculate System (MARS), which is a blood-purification system based on albumin dialysis, which includes a charcoal filter. This liver support system utilizes an albumin-enriched dialysate to facilitate removal of albumin-bound toxins. The patient in this case report was a 45-year-old male in status epilepticus, who received high dose intravenous phenytoin and later developed acute rhabdomyolysis leading to acute renal failure, which lead further to higher drug accumulation. The patient developed altered mental status and remained unconscious for more than 8 days despite enteral activated charcoal treatment and continuous venous hemofiltration. Throughout his stay, his liver enzymes started to elevate signifying hepatotoxicity and was noted to have multiple rounds of tachyarrhythmias (ventricular tachycardia) and bradyarrhythmias, requiring temporary cardiac pacing, indicating cardiotoxicity. During the treatment with MARS, they measured total and free phenytoin levels from four segments of the MARS circuit: before, twice during and once at the end of the treatment. The treatment lasted a total of 11.5 hours. Once results were obtained, the authors reported a linear and rapid decrease of both total and free serum phenytoin concentration (from 32 to 11 micrometer and 9.8 to 2.0 micrometer, respectively) throughout the treatment. They also concluded that not only did MARS reduce phenytoin from the blood, but it also removed the free radicals created by phenytoin which can lead to oxidative stress in the patient. [23]

In another case report, in a critically ill patient who was found to have falsely therapeutic phenytoin levels due to hypoalbuminemia, the patient received high-flux dialysis and charcoal hemoperfusion, which resulted in significant decrease in total phenytoin levels by the third day of treatment. [24] It has been shown that patients on chronic hemodialysis and who are on phenytoin management for seizures, require a dose of phenytoin after their dialysis treatment to prevent seizures, due to increased removal of free phenytoin from high-flux dialysis. Patients on chronic dialysis have increased free phenytoin in the body due to phenytoin being displaced from serum proteins secondary to competitive binding of uremic toxins. [25] So, the authors hypothesized that this mechanism of increased free phenytoin levels in dialysis patients can be mirrored in patients with hypoalbuminemia and thus can be treated with high-flux dialysis to lower free serum levels of phenytoin. [24] Hemodialysis can be done by low flux or high flux membrane. High-flux dialysis is defined as a $\beta 2$-microglobulin clearance of over 20 ml/min. High flux membranes compared to low flux have larger pores and allow diffusion of greater amounts of uremic toxins. Low-flux hemodialysis has not been shown to reduce phenytoin levels significantly, due to phenytoin's high protein binding. [14] Thus, weighing the available evidence, extracorporeal removal of phenytoin is rarely needed, but can be considered in severe cases and with guidelines published by the EXTRIP group as discussed above.

If the Purple Glove Syndrome (PGS) develops in a patient receiving intravenous phenytoin while in the hospital setting the treatment is mainly supportive with cessation of the medication, elevation of the limb, application of warm compresses and analgesia, such as anti-inflammatories. [26,27] One case reported adequate analgesia and full recovery of a patient's hand within a month with the use of continuous blockade of the patient's brachial plexus with a low concentration of bupivacaine and fentanyl. [28] A second case report showed adequate pain relief as well with a brachial plexus block, when conventional oral NSAIDs failed. [29] It is unknown what causes the syndrome at this time, but the main theory is that it is due to the extravasation of medication causing swelling, pain, and discoloration of the extremity distal to the site of where the medication is being administered. Although even rarer, PGS has also been seen in oral administration of phenytoin, but the treatment is the same. [26] Most cases of PGS resolve within days to weeks, with rare development of complications such as ulcers, necrosis, ischemia, or compartment syndrome. If such complications do occur, consultation with a surgeon would be advised. [30]

As mentioned, fosphenytoin is the more water-soluble prodrug of phenytoin that is metabolized by phosphatases to yield phenytoin and inorganic phosphate. Theoretically, the generation of inorganic phosphate during this conversion can bind calcium, which could alter cardiac conduction as a result of the indirectly induced hypocalcemia. One case reports a 23-year-old male patient with an untreated seizure disorder who developed prolongation of the ST segment and QT interval as well as merging of the P and T wave after administration of fosphenytoin, 1500mg phenytoin equivalents over 85 minutes. These ECG findings were consistent with hypocalcemia. The patient was normocalcemic prior to the medication administration, with measured plasma total calcium level of 9.5 mg/dL. He was then noted to have decreased total and ionized serum calcium concentrations after medication administration, with serum total calcium level measured at 7.5 mg/dL and an ionized calcium level of 4.52 mg/dL. A serum phenytoin level was also measured and found to be supratherapeutic at 16.2 mg/L. There were no hemodynamic compromise to the decrease in calcium concentration and the ECG normalized. [31]

The disposition of the patient and decision to admit largely depends on the clinical scenario of the toxicity. In patients where there are significant neurological manifestations such as altered mental status or ataxia, fall precautions should be instituted and the patient would not be considered safe to discharge home. On the contrary, a bedbound patient with modestly elevated phenytoin concentration may be discharged with close follow up. All patients who are admitted to the hospital require frequent neurological checks regardless of the route of overdose, whether oral or intravenous. Cardiac monitoring on the other hand is only required for those rare patients with intravenous overdoses who develop cardiac manifestations. [17]

## Conclusion

There should be a high index of suspicion when diagnosing toxicity from phenytoin, which is made easier by specific physical exam manifestations, specifically neurological abnormalities such as nystagmus and ataxia. Concentrations of the drug can assist in the diagnosis and management of toxicity, but must be corrected for patients with low protein binding capabilities. Although treatment remains largely supportive, MDAC can be used in certain populations in order to enhance its elimination. The role for HD in phenytoin poisoned patient is dependent on the clinical picture, with the EXTRIP workgroup providing evidence based recommendations. Disposition depends on the clinical scenario of toxicity, with frequent neurologic assessments required, but cardiac monitoring is rarely needed.

## References

[1] Wyte CD, Berk WA. Severe oral phenytoin overdose does not cause cardiovascular morbidity. *Ann Emerg Med.* 1991; 20(5):508-12.

[2] Su CM, Kung CT, Wang YC, Lu CH. Life-threatening cardiotoxicity due to chronic oral phenytoin overdose. *Neurol India.* 2009; 57(2):200-2.

[3] Srinivasan G, Wyawahare M, Mathen PG, Subrahmanyam DK. Life-threatening bradyarrhythmia with oral phenytoin overdose. *J Pharmacol Pharmacother.* 2015; 6(3):179-81.

[4] Nitya R: Cerebellar degeneration following long-term phenytoin therapy. *Neurology.* 1976 September; 26 (9): 818

[5] Goldfrank L. *Goldfrank's Toxicologic emergencies.* (2019). 11ed. New York. McGraw-Hill.

[6] Lindow J. Phenytoin toxicity associated with hypoalbumemia in critically ill patients. *Chest.* 1994 Feb; 105 (2): 602-4.

[7] Cadle RM, Zenon G. Fluconazole-induced symptomatic phenytoin toxicity. *Annals of Pharmacotherapy.* 1994.

[8] Pollack T, Slayter K. Hazards of doubling phenytoin dose in the face of an unrecognized interaction with ciprofloxacin. *Annals of Pharmacotherapy.* 1997.

[9] Antoniou T, Gomes T. Trimethoprim/Sulframethoxazole- induced phenytoin toxicity in the elderly: a population based study. *Brit Jour of Clin. Pharmacology.* Vol 71. Issue 4. 2010.

[10] Marin L, Garcia-Penas J. Phenytoin-induced visual disturbances mimicking Delirium Tremens in a child. *European Journal of Pediatric Neurology.* 2010. Vol 14.issue5, 460-463.

[11] Shores MM, Sloan KL. Phenytoin-induced visual disturbances misdiagnosed as alcohol withdrawal. *Psychosomatics.* 2002; 43(4):335-6.

[12] Katz A, Hoffman R. Phenytoin toxicity from smoking crack cocaine adultered with phenytoin. *Annals of Emergency medicine.* 1993.

[13] Polman A.J. Early – onset phenytoin toxicity mimicking a renopulmonary syndrome. *European Respiratory Journal.* 1998; 11:501-503.

[14] Agrawal M, Borkar SA. Phenytoin Toxicity manifesting as acute psychosis: An uncommon side effect of a common drug. *Asian Journal of Neurosurgery.* 2019 Apr-Jun; 14 (2): 532-534.

[15] Wen-Hung Chung et al. Genetic Variants Associated with Phenytoin-Related Severe Cutaneous Adverse Reaction. *JAMA.* 2014; 312(5):525-534.

[16] Craig S. Phenytoin overdose complicated by prolonged intoxication and residual neurological deficits. *Emerg Med Australas.* 2004; 16(4):361-5.

[17] Stilman N, Masdeu JC. Incidence of seizures with phenytoin toxicity. *Neurology*. 1985; 35:1769–1772.

[18] Craig, S. (2005). *Phenytoin Poisoning. Neurocritical Care,* 3(2), 161–170. doi: 10.1385/ncc:3:2:161

[19] Guldiken B, Rémi J, Noachtar S. Cardiovascular adverse effects of phenytoin. *J Neurol.* 2016; 263(5):861-870.

[20] Evers ML, Izhar A, Aqil A. Cardiac monitoring after phenytoin overdose. *Heart Lung.* 1997; 26(4):325-8.

[21] Iorga A, Horowitz BZ. *Phenytoin Toxicity.* [Updated 2019 Feb 28]. In: StatPearls. Treasure Island (FL): StatPearls Publishing; 2019 Jan.

[22] Skinner CG, Chang AS, Matthews AS, Reedy SJ, Morgan BW. Randomized controlled study on the use of multiple-dose activated charcoal in patients with supratherapeutic phenytoin levels. *Clin Toxicol (Phila).* 2012; 50(8):764-9.

[23] Anseeuw K, Mowry JB, Burdmann EA, Ghannoum M, Hoffman RS, Gosselin S, Lavergne V, Nolin TD; EXTRIP Workgroup. (2016) "Extracorporeal Treatment in Phenytoin Poisoning: Systematic Review and Recommendations from the EXTRIP (Extracorporeal Treatments in Poisoning) Workgroup." *Am J Kidney Dis.* 67(2):187-97.

[24] Sen S, Ratnaraj N, Davies NA, et al. Treatment of phenytoin toxicity by the molecular adsorbents recirculating system (MARS). *Epilepsia.* 2003; 44(2):265-7.

[25] De schoenmakere G, De waele J, Terryn W, et al. Phenytoin intoxication in critically ill patients. *Am J Kidney Dis.* 2005; 45(1):189-92.

[26] Frenchie D, Bastani B. Significant removal of phenytoin during high flux dialysis with cellulose triacetate dialyzer. *Nephrol Dial Transplant.* 1998; 13(3):817-8.

[27] Jain RS, Nagpal K, Kumar S, Prakash S, Handa R. Purple glove syndrome occurring after oral administration of phenytoin in therapeutic doses: Mechanism still a dilemma. *Am J Emerg Med.* 2015; 33(1):123.e5-6.

[28] Newman JW, Blunck JR, Fields RK, Croom JE. Fosphenytoin-induced purple glove syndrome: A case report. *Clin Neurol Neurosurg.* 2017; 160:50-53.

[29] Singh G, Cherian VT, Thomas BP. Low-concentration, continuous brachial plexus block in the management of Purple Glove Syndrome: a case report. *J Med Case Rep.* 2010; 4:48.

[30] Senthilkumaran S, Balamurgan N, Suresh P, Thirumalaikolundusubramanian P. Purple glove syndrome: A looming threat. *J Neurosci Rural Pract.* 2010; 1(2):121-2.

[31] Chokshi R, Openshaw J, Mehta NN, Mohler E. Purple glove syndrome following intravenous phenytoin administration. *Vasc Med.* 2007; 12(1):29-31.

[32] Keegan MT, Bondy LR, Blackshear JL, Lanier WL. Hypocalcemia-like electrocardiographic changes after administration of intravenous fosphenytoin. *Mayo Clin Proc.* 2002; 77(6):584-6.

# ABOUT THE EDITOR

*Payal Sud* is a double-board certified Emergency Medicine Physician and Medical Toxicologist. She serves as the Associate Chairperson of Emergency Medicine at Glen Cove Hospital, a part of the Northwell Health System. She is also an Assistant Professor of Emergency Medicine at the Zucker School of Medicine at Hofstra/Northwell. Additionally, she is intimately involved in the education of the Medical Toxicology fellows at North Shore University Hospital.

Besides her interests in Medical Toxicology, Dr. Sud is involved in several initiatives to improve the care of patients with acute strokes as well as patients with sepsis in the Emergency Department. She is currently actively involved in improving patient experience and palliative care in the Emergency Department through a multi-disciplinary approach.

# INDEX

## E



## F

## K



## L



## M



## N



## O

## S



## T

## U



## V



## W



## X